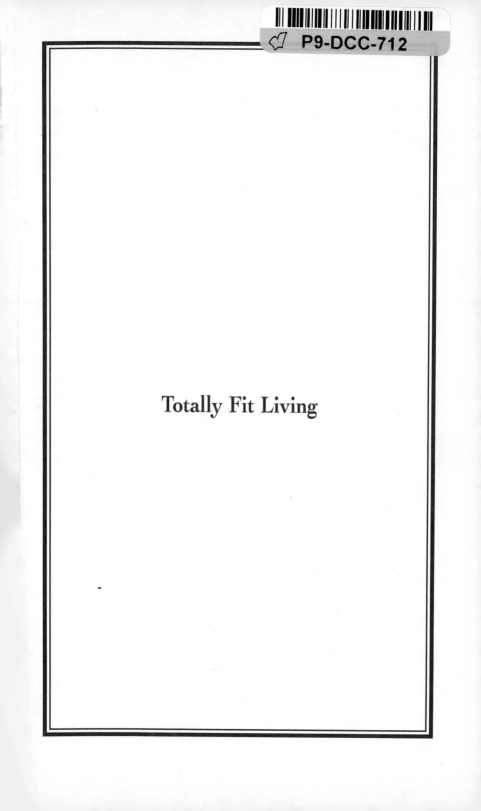

Totally Fit Living

Totally Fit Living

A 30-Day Program for Total Health & Happiness

ROBERT KRONEMEYER, Ph.D.

Health Communications, Inc.
Deerfield Beach, Florida

Library of Congress Cataloging-in-Publication Data

Kronemeyer, Robert.
    [Syntonics]
        Totally fit living : a 30-day program for total health &
    happiness / Robert Kronemeyer.
            p. cm.
        Originally published: Syntonics. Englewood Cliffs, N.J. :
    Prentice Hall, ©1994.
        Includes bibliographical references and index.
        ISBN 1-55874-396-0 (trade paper)
        1. Self-actualization (Psychology) 2. Happiness. 3. Health.
    I. Title.
    [BF637.S4K76   1996]
    158'.1--dc20   96-14527
                                                                CIP

©1994, 1996 Robert Kronemeyer
ISBN 1-55874-396-0

Publisher: Health Communications, Inc.
            3201 S.W. 15th Street
            Deerfield Beach, Florida 33442-8190

Cover design by Lawna Patterson Oldfield

DEDICATION

To patients of physicians
> who realize that drugs and surgery remove no cause and
> who seek the knowledge to prevent further illness and to
> build wellness

To patients of therapists and psychiatrists
> who realize that talking and tranquilizing are not enough
> and who seek a healthy lifestyle and dynamic therapy

To doctors of all varieties
> who wish better health for their patients and themselves
> and who realize the need for a wholistic approach to health

To educators
> who realize that self-fulfillment stems from self-knowl-
> edge and self-discipline and who seek this creative path
> for themselves and their students

To parents
> who can admit the truth that the best way to help their
> children grow is to improve themselves — their physical,
> emotional, mental, and spiritual aliveness

To all those
    who want vitality instead of fatigue, relaxation instead
of stress, healing instead of drugging, joy instead of
heaviness, love instead of fear, and wholeness instead of
separation

CONTENTS

**Chapter Thirteen: The Syntonic View of
Healthy Spirituality**

Chapter Fourteen: Improve Your Spiritual Health

Chapter Fifteen: Your Greatest Opportunity for Personal Growth

CHARTS

ACKNOWLEDGMENTS

So many people have helped me in my search for knowledge and wisdom. In particular I extend my heartfelt gratitude to:

My mother Dorothy and my father Ferdinand; Dr. Donald Papon and Rex Hearn who were with me from the beginning; Bob Silverstein, agent extraordinaire whose wit and wisdom were unfailing; editors Doug Corcoran and Barbara O'Brien whose suggestions and faith were invaluable; my teachers at Amherst College, Union Theological Seminary, and Columbia University; Dr. Wilhelm Reich, Dr. Theodor Reik, Dr. Harry Bone, Dr. Alexander Lowen, Dr. John Pierrakos, Dr. Kilton Stewart, Dr. Alan Cott, Dr. Alexander Wolf, and Dr. Fritz Perls, all of whom helped in my personal growth and clinical expertise; Zen master George Ohsawa (macrobiotics), 9th Dan master Koichi Tohei (aikido), Swami Satchidananda (yoga) and Maharishi Mahesh Yogi; my friend Karan Singh, Maharajah of Kashmir whose warmth and wisdom inspired me; wholistic colleagues and leading nutritional and complementary physicians in New York City Dr. Azim Etemadi, Dr. Robert

C. Atkins, Dr. Robert Wallis, and Dr. Stuart Berger; Dr. Julian Whitaker of Newport Beach, California; and my son Jeff, for his faith and love, and for creating with Elyn, Jessica, and Olivia the happy democratic family which is the essential foundation for a healthy society and a sane world.

And to my patients who taught me so much—and in becoming well in body, emotions, mind, and spirit, after failing in more partial therapies, validated my faith in the total Syntonic Therapy and bio-neural re-programming herein described.

Spiritually I have a deep bond with Hippocrates who taught that "a wise man should consider that health is the greatest of human blessings"; with the Delphic Oracle who counseled "Know Thyself"; with Jesus who revealed that "Love casts out fear", and with Rabindranath Tagore whose *Gitanjali* (song offerings to God) can melt the hardest heart and free mankind from the alienation of atheism and agnosticism, since "Only the pure in heart see God."

Lastly, as one infinitesimal particle in the Infinite, I thank what Albert Einstein called "that supreme reasoning power which is revealed in the incomprehensible universe and forms my idea of God." That Life Force is not only transcendent but also immanent and within. As a verse from one of the Vedas says: "The inner intelligence of the body is the ultimate and supreme genius in nature. It mirrors the wisdom of the cosmos."

INTRODUCTION

Syntonics is a practical way of achieving the health and happiness that is our birthright and that we all seek. The natural state of syntony or harmony is experienced as we bring together *("syn")* a relaxed body, positive emotions, constructive thoughts, and a bright spirit. We will then know that flow of positive energy *("tony")* that is the source of self-esteem, joy, and freedom. Syntony is the richness of feeling that gives life meaning, purpose, and value. (This is described as the Self in the Personality Chart on page xiii.) Sadly, most human beings fail in this pursuit. The staggering cost of health care and hospitals, drugs, and surgery leaves no family untouched.

Happily, the good news is that in these pages you will find the practical way to *prevent* physical, emotional, mental, and psychosomatic illness by living in syntony with nature. And as a bonus, in so doing your "inner physician" will cure many of the symptoms and illnesses you have brought on yourself already. Would you like the glowing health, pain-free life, and dynamic vigor that you were designed for?

Happiness also seems to elude most people—rich and poor alike. Thoreau observed that most people live lives of "quiet desperation." But Syntonics will also show you the less traveled road that leads to happiness, peace of mind, and self-fulfillment. Of course, these are qualities of body, emotions, mind, and soul that cannot be bought at any price. How, then, can one attain them?

Here is where you come in. You can choose to read this book and put it aside with all the others, or use it as the most exciting challenge you have ever faced to re-create your life in a practical, day-by-day program of *your own creation!* I will be your guide, but you must climb the mountain. I will outline specific ways for you to improve all four aspects of your being—your body, emotions, mind, and spirit. These ways are taken from Eastern wisdom and Western science and are guaranteed to yield positive results. Do we not reap as we sow?

How to Use This Book to Fulfill Your Life

Do you remember the Sufi story of the blind men who came upon an elephant in the forest? Each one touched a part of the beast and thought the whole animal was like a serpent (the trunk), a tree (the leg), a wall (the side), and a rope (the tail).

Just as an elephant is more than the sum of its parts, we human beings are more than the sum of our four aspects— our physical, emotional, mental, and spiritual dimensions. The goal of Syntonics is to strengthen the health of all four of these aspects so that together they can be synthesized into a complete and fulfilled person. All are interrelated and each will affect the others. Thus, ancient wisdom stressed a "sound mind in a sound body," called the body the "temple of the spirit," (I Corinthians 6:19) and reminded us that "out of the heart are the issues of life." (Proverbs 4:23)

Do you agree with me that no one can change or improve your life but you? If so, as you read this total program to re-create your life, take notes as you go along, so you will have the excitement of planning the things that you decide to try in your new lifestyle.

Section I deals with your body. Note the foods and supplements you choose to eat, and take time out to eliminate junk foods from your cupboard (sugar, white rice, salt, white flour products, margarine, etc.). Write down the new way of low-fat eating that will do wonders for your body, with new menus you wish to try. Include in your personal program a schedule for fasting (perhaps one day a week on vegetable juice), exercise, rest, and the elimination of toxic habits. Also make a special "start the day" program for yourself that includes breathing and tension release exercises. Later you can add emotional release and meditation techniques.

While reading Section II on your emotions, practice using sound and movements to release tensions or held-in emotions you are aware of or just to express exuberance if you feel great at the moment. Perhaps you will want to use the power of positive anger to challenge fears or sad feelings that have held you back in your life. Write down the techniques that work for you, and after you release negative feelings, practice positive imagery to build positive emotions. Then choose the steps to emotional health that are of most help to you.

In Section III you have a great opportunity to change "old records" from the past that have had a negative effect on your freedom and self-esteem. Most are negative "old baggage" from parents and teachers that have to be thrown out. Write down these destructive attitudes and beliefs, and next to each one write down a rational and positive statement that contradicts it. Think of these negative attitudes as part of your fearful, negative, and hurt "inner child." Hold a pillow, representing your inner child, and in a firm and loving way tell your inner child that you are taking over as a good parent and helping your child change and grow. Finally, review the steps to overcoming negative thinking that you want to include in your program.

In Section IV on your spirit, practice the meditation techniques and the deep breathing that will help you experience the cosmic and inner power we call God. Only when the spirit flows through a relaxed and healthy body, with an open heart and a peaceful mind, do we experience freedom and joy. In religious terms, it is written in the Scriptures: "The Lord is the Spirit and where the Spirit of the Lord is, there is freedom." (II Corinthians 3:17) Also see which of the "deadly sins" are disturbing your life, and after rising to a higher level of consciousness through meditation, visualize yourself caught in that particular trap. Continually seeing this through the eyes of your higher Self will bring about spiritual healing.

Now review your notes and draw up your own program to start the day. Next, outline a plan of action to deal with any exceptional stress that comes into your life. (Remember, we cannot control what happens to us at times, but we can learn to control how we react to these events.) Next, draw up an overall Syntonic program for your new lifestyle for health and happiness. Lastly, write down positive affirmations about your Self and positive beliefs that come from your heart and spirit. Even better, put them on a tape and play them back to yourself before you go to sleep, so that positive energy can continue healing your whole being during the night.

Appendix I will show you the democratic way to a happy family. Folks, we have the best philosophy in the world. You will see miracles happen when parents and children share their hurts and their joy and grow in honesty and respect. And spread the good news! Encourage your friends to benefit as well.

Appendix II works like magic to improve any relationship between two people who are willing to give it a try. I have seen the empathy exercise save marriages and families where all else failed. And why not? Empathy is love in action; and love is the highest power in the world.

Appendix III lists nutrients which, when used to replace the high-fat and "refined" junk food diet of America, could save us from being one of the sickest countries in the world. Start with yourself—the proof is in the pudding!

Appendix IV presents a far more important challenge than having an American suburb on Mars. The three R's are important, but obviously not enough. Our schools create new hordes to fill our hospitals, jails, divorce courts, and welfare programs. Creative growth groups would teach, in practice, the fourth R: respect for oneself, for others, for one's body, mind, and spirit, and for life itself. Schools could be places where self-knowledge and mutual understanding replace violence and fear. Help get a pilot program going!

Appendix V is yet another opportunity to stem the drugging epidemic—the myth of the Magic Pill—that is creating the fastest growing malady in the world—iatrogenic (doctor- and drug-caused) disease.

I know how much the Syntonic way did to improve my health and happiness, and naturally, my friend, I want the

same for you. Imagine yourself with a healthy and vigorous
body; an open heart that loves yourself, others, and the
Higher Power; a mind that is free to think clearly or to be
peaceful and not think if you choose; and a rejuvenated
spirit that can enjoy faith, hope, and love.

Here's the chance of a lifetime to make the most of all the
gifts you have been given. With purpose, planning, and perseverance, you can find the meaning of your life; you can
scale your own Mt. Everest and become your real Self as
described in the Personality Chart on page xxvi.

How to Use the Personality Chart

Think of this chart as a map of your inner universe. On
the right is a description of the way we are meant to be
according to the plan of the Great Designer. Hopefully you
have at least glimpsed what it is like to experience that natural and healthy state I call the Self. Is it not awesome to
realize that these billions of cells of which we are composed
are meant to work together in a Syntonic way to fulfill our
potential in all four dimensions of our life? In this state, in
which the parasympathetic nervous system is in effect, we
are in peace and harmony with ourselves and with the universe. In its fullest flower, this experience is called Oneness,
Heaven, or Enlightenment.

Ancient wisdom taught that proper care of and respect
for one's body was the foundation of this state of syntony
and well-being. Thus, as you choose the changes you decide
to make in your own life from the first four chapters on the
human body, you will start to strengthen the foundation of
your being. As you change your lifestyle in a healthier direction through improved nutrition, eliminating poisons from

your body, healthy breathing, prudent exercise, deep relaxation, and self-reflexology, you will also be enhancing your emotions, mind, and spirit.

The healthy Self is emotionally positive, as the chart describes, and loving and courageous. In contrast, the disturbed, anxious state (the sympathetic nervous system) is designed to help us face and/or escape danger. Facing a robber or a hurricane, we become ready to react in a fight-or-flight manner, and when the threat is over, hopefully return to the positive state. However, here's the rub: From unnatural and violent childbirth, through infancy and childhood (that often lack, in varying degrees, the love, respect, and security so essential to emotional health), many become chronically geared to the anxious, conflicted, fight-or-flight state. In extremes, this makes life a living hell for the hapless person.

Do fear, anger, and sadness take most of your emotional energy? Were you punished for expressing these emotions? As you read Section II, write down the methods you can use to regain your positive emotions. Psychoanalyzing can reveal how you were hurt but does not usually cure the problem. The good news is that using the Personality Chart and these specific techniques, you can change in the present and renew the positive feelings you are meant to enjoy.

Next note that in the healthy state we are meant to be mentally clear, honest, and rational. Is your mind, however, still playing "old records" that are self-punishing? Write them down, and next to them write contradicting rational thoughts. Then choose from the chart the main defenses you have used to deal with your inner negativity and with your fear of the outer world. By using the techniques in Section III, you will be able to cancel the negative thoughts that are part of these defenses that limit your freedom. As you work on eliminating the irrational thoughts that accompany these bogus attitudes and replace them with honest and rational thoughts, the truth will "set you free." The Self is not fearful and negative in thought and action! Such effort will be more valuable in making positive changes in your life than years of passive analyzing on an expensive couch.

Perhaps you have a friend or several friends who are also seeking a happier and less traveled path. Meeting together and sharing the journey could make it even more meaningful and exciting.

Lastly, the Personality Chart describes the healthy spiritual state as being in touch with the Life Force of the universe. Whether a person belongs to a particular religion or not, the test of true spirituality is in the capacity of the person to experience syntony (the sum of all of the person's parts into a creative wholeness). Positive energy, love, is the binding power that enables us to feel at one with our Self, with others, and with the Creator. Where this spirit is lacking, religion becomes a farce.

Note that where there is syntony and wholeness, the negative emotions — the neurotic defenses, the symptoms of disease, and the muscular tension — all dissolve like clouds in the face of the sun. We are made of stardust and spirit and ultimately can only find inner peace when we regain our Oneness with the Source of our being.

With this in mind, write down the methods in Section IV that you are willing to practice to regain your syntony and freedom from fear and alienation.

Bear in mind that the Self on the Personality Chart is our natural and undisturbed state. There will be times when we will experience fear, sadness, and assertive anger, and appropriately so. But practicing the Syntonic way will prevent you from getting *stuck* in negativity when life is nasty, brutish, and short. Pulling the weeds and cultivating the garden makes it all worthwhile!

Affirmations and visualizations based on the Personality Chart can be a valuable part of your self-transformation. Here is a sample which you can use, change, and add to as you wish, and also record to play back to yourself.

My natural state is to be whole and free.

My body is a miraculous, self-healing creation.

I am responsible for my own health or illness.

I can regain a healthy and relaxed body.

My emotions are meant to be positive and enjoyable.

I can learn to let go of anxious and negative feelings.

I can use my anger as a positive force for inner growth.

Loving myself, others, and the Creator is my strength.

My thoughts determine my feelings and actions.

I can reject negative thoughts and choose constructive ones.

In meditation I can find peace of mind beyond thought.

In syntony with God, defenses and the deadly sins melt away.

The more I lose my ego, the more I find my Self.

I picture myself in vibrant physical health.

I picture myself warm, loving, and compassionate.

I picture myself free of negative thoughts and defenses.

I picture my soul constantly restored by the Holy Spirit.

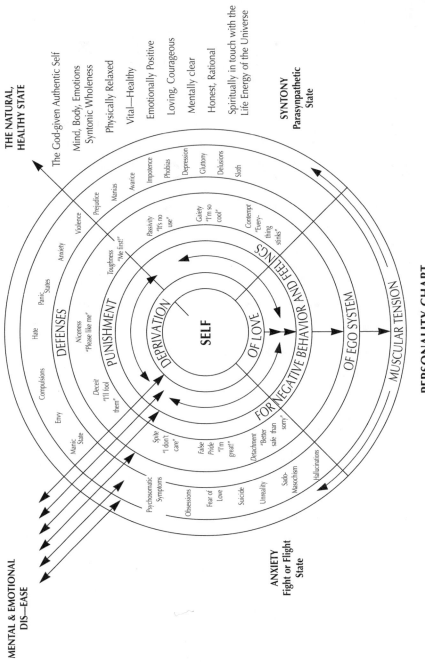

PERSONALITY CHART

THE PERSONALITY CHART

THE SELF: The undisturbed state of the healthy infant and the mature and loving adult

DEPRIVATION OF LOVE: The needs of infants for nursing and love are seldom satisfied and lay the groundwork for disturbed emotions, thoughts, and behavior.

FEAR, ANGER, AND DEPRESSION: This "unholy trinity" is caused by inadequate nursing, closeness, warmth, and love. These negative emotions and abnormal physical tensions are created in the insecure infant and child who forms a "fear bond" with the mother.

PUNISHMENT FOR NEGATIVE BEHAVIOR AND FEELINGS: Lacking education for parenthood, parents frequently repeat the same negative reactions and punishments that they received from their parents. The child is deprived of the understanding and loving discipline that he or she needs to develop trust and self-esteem.

THE NINE NEUROTIC CHARACTER ATTITUDES: These defensive attitudes are developed in childhood, as the child seeks to deal with the painful emotions of fear, anger, and sadness and the guilt he or she is made to feel for having these natural reactions. At the same time that these attitudes are self-protective, they are also self-crippling and often provoke further punishment.

THE DEFENSES OF THE EGO SYSTEM: Although these defenses result in neurotic safety and satisfaction, they keep the individual caught in his or her armor and separated from the positive core of the loving, rational, and assertive Self.

THE SYMPTOMS OF EMOTIONAL AND MENTAL DIS-EASE: These are the symptoms that plague individual and social health and harmony. They are contagious and will continue to undermine civilization until humans learn to understand and respect the physical, emotional, mental, and spiritual laws of the universe.

The Human Body

The doctor of the future
will give no medicine, but will
interest his patients in the care of
the human frame and diet, and
the cause and prevention
of disease.

—THOMAS A. EDISON

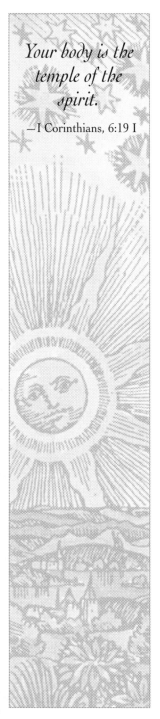

Your body is the temple of the spirit.

—I Corinthians, 6:19 I

ONE

The Many Benefits of Syntonics

Both Prevention and Cure

We are in the beginning of a health revolution. A new level of health consciousness is becoming prevalent among some doctors and laypeople alike. The realization is dawning that health cannot be dispensed by electronic gadgets, elaborate hospitals, "gold-plated" stethoscopes, or new chemical concoctions. Though medical intervention is necessary in acute illnesses, the real task is to prevent disease and to build health. Health is

3

not merely an absence of symptoms, but a vital state of well-being in all areas of one's life.

The plague of degenerative diseases such as cancer, heart disease, lung disease, stroke, ulcers, alimentary malfunctions, arthritis, and diabetes is human-made and largely preventable. Syntonics can prevent and—when not too far gone—cure these degenerative diseases by eliminating high fat, processed and refined foods, smoking, lethargy, obesity, sugar, salt, alcohol, and caffeine. A healthy, cleansing, and energy-creating diet of complex carbohydrates (fruits, vegetables, and whole grains) with essential roughage and fiber will shorten the transit time of waste through the body and lessen the buildup of cholesterol. Is it not ironic that the father of medicine, Hippocrates, said: "Let your food be your medicine," whereas most physicians, even today, are only aware of medications (with often damaging side effects) and surgery (which is often unnecessary) and are ignorant about nutritional healing by creating health?

A notable exception is David Reuben, M.D. who recommends "high fiber protection from six of the most serious diseases of civilization:

- cancer of the colon and rectum;
- heart attack causing 700,000 deaths in America each year;
- diverticulosis, a disease of the colon affecting almost half the population over forty;
- appendicitis, the primary abdominal surgical emergency, causing 200,000 operations and 20,000 deaths each year;
- obesity which handicaps twenty-five percent of our citizens; and
- hemorrhoids, constipation and varicose veins, those annoying legacies of civilization." [1]

[1] David Reuben, M.D., *Everything You Always Wanted To Know About Nutrition*, Avon Press, N.Y., 1979, p. 28.

Groups who avoid red meat, coffee, alcohol, and tobacco such as the Seventh-Day Adventists, according to a study by Dr. David Snowden for the National Institute of Health, were found to have a much lower incidence[2] of all these diseases and live seven years longer than the average American. A study of their whole way of life is typical of the wholistic approach of the "new" doctor.

One such physician, Bruce Halstead, M.D., interpreted the results of this study as follows:

> Analyses of their life style reveal that Adventists tend toward a vegetarian diet, abstain from caffeinated drinks and smoking, and eat less junk foods. The endorsement of certain spiritual values is also believed to be an important factor. . . . [I]t is this composite which leads one to the proposition that a [w]wholistic approach to metabolic therapy has merit.[3]

Dr. Halstead also points out the resistance on the part of the general medical population to a prevention approach to health care: "After all, you don't make much money by keeping people healthy. Moreover it's hard on the pharmaceutical industry, and even worse if we don't keep those hospital beds full. A healthy society could bring about a sick medical economy."

The wholistic approach to health is concerned with removing the causes of illness rather than treating the symptoms with drugs and/or surgery. A garden may look good if the weeds are cut down, but weeds soon grow again

---

[2] Jane E. Brody, "Adventists Are Gold Mine for Research on Disease," *The New York Times*, Nov. 11, 1986, p. 10.

[3] *The Journal of the International Academy of Nutritional Consultants*, Vol. I, No. 3.

unless their roots are eliminated. An acquaintance of mine had bypass surgery because residues were blocking the vessels bringing blood to his heart. While recovering at the hospital, he was served the same high-fat and "refined" foods that led to his illness; and he was not given any guidance about preventing a recurrence of this condition. Five years later, he was forced to undergo the expensive trauma of further surgery.

Since the time of Louis Pasteur, medicine has been preoccupied with battling microscopic organisms that are harmful to the human body. Yet we all have observed that some people exposed to communicable diseases contract them while others do not. We correctly say that the latter "have greater resistance," but what is resistance? An organism with a higher degree of vitality and greater health has more adequate defense mechanisms as well as a better biochemical balance, due primarily to superior nutrition. Syntonics will show you how to increase your vitality.

This view is espoused by another outstanding wholistic physician, H. Ray Evers, M.D., who has successfully treated thousands of cases of "incurable" degenerative diseases when conventional medical approaches have failed. Dr. Evers's clinical experience has led him to believe that malnutrition (the ordinary American diet) is the cause of acute or communicable illnesses as well as the slower and more insidious variety—the degenerative illnesses common in industrial societies.

In explaining the cause of illnesses, Dr. Evers parts company with the mainstream of thought derived from Pasteur:

Although I realize that my view in this regard is on a collision course with Pasteur's concept of germs causing disease

I cannot accept a premise that is alien to my own experience. This obvious controversial stance requires elaboration. I do not repudiate the fact that germs can and do contribute to disease. However I am convinced that germs are only disease causing in the absence of proper bio-chemical balance which is precipitated by malnutrition. Therefore I am relegating germs to the number three position in the progression of causes of disease and ranking malnutrition and biochemical imbalance as one and two respectively.[4]

You Are What You Eat

Proper nutrition is essential both to clear out residues in the circulatory system and to nourish properly the sixty trillion cells of the body, which miraculously accomplish the thousands of chemical reactions integral to the maintenance of health. Unless the system is relatively unobstructed, many of those cells will become toxic and prey to disease. Once patients have been treated in this fashion, it is imperative that they remain on a maintenance program of good nutrition to avoid a recurrence of the illness. The proverb "you are what you eat" is valid, for in the final analysis, the nature of the ingested food determines the accumulation of residue in the vascular system.

Most of us, whether doctors or therapists or laypeople, have been taught to "do something" when symptoms appear, such as taking pills, drugs, or even undergoing surgery. We have been educated away from considering another alternative to treating symptoms. I agree with Dr. Robert Mendelsohn's statement that "if 90 percent of the doctoring going on were to stop, we'd be much better off . . . [M]ore people die of legally prescribed valium than from illegal

---

[4] Ibid.

heroin." The pills sold to doctors by competitive drug companies often have side-effects worse than the symptoms they were meant to cure. Dr. Mendelsohn indicts modern medicine for the "ritual mutilations" of often unnecessary surgery, and he calls the New (wholistic) Doctor one who acknowledges "nature as the prime healer":

> Instead of viewing the patient as a collection of symptoms localized in a single spot, the New Doctor will see the whole person as a context and possible cause for disease. . . . Since he will reject much of modern medicine's machinery, he will be knowledgeable in unorthodox methods of treating disease, including nutritional therapy, acupuncture, kinesiology, chiropractic, homeopathy and others.[5]

The New Doctor will teach people how to keep themselves healthy and how to restore health and balance without the aid of a professional. Dr. Mendelsohn and other spiritually minded colleagues are introducing a New Medical School designed to teach physicians not "to subdue . . . rather to restore the balance of Nature." In the legacy of Hippocrates, they will take seriously the injunction of the Hippocratic Oath: *"First, do no harm."*

Herman's Hemmorhoids

Herman is a perfect example of a patient being seen as a symptom, rather than as a whole human being. He came to me for Syntonic therapy through a friend who had been helped. He was an older man concerned about being depressed, anxious, and always worried. When he mentioned an impending hemmorhoid

---

[5] Robert Mendelsohn, M.D., *Confessions of a Medical Heretic*, Contemporary Books, Inc., Chicago, 1979.

operation, my ears tingled. I had just read about an unscrupulous segment of physicians and unnecessary surgery being performed on trusting women (i.e., a billion dollars taken literally at knife point, in one year, for *unnecessary* Caesarians, which deprive mother and infant of a natural and healthy birth experience).

I told Herman I had helped others avoid the surgery he had been "sold," and I gained his cooperation. Within a month of eliminating fatty and fried foods, white flour, and pastries, while adding fruit, vegetables, and whole grains (which are full of essential fiber for proper elimination), Herman no longer needed the surgery. More importantly, his chance of avoiding more serious illnesses improved with better functioning (cancer of the colon, heart disease, etc., of which the hemmorhoid symptom was only a sign). I imagined the spirit of Hippocrates smiling happily. . . .

Being Your Own Doctor

How can a person maintain his or her own health? By leading a meaningful life in which proper nutrition, physical exercise, and stress management combine with an appropriate balance of love, play, and work. Such rational goals call for a revamping of our educational systems as well. For example, school lunches should provide daily examples of whole natural foods and a context in which students can practice ways of building health as well as learning algebra. Likewise, the classroom should teach self-knowledge and emotional growth through group interaction, as well as instructing students in the rules of grammar; and compassion and helpfulness toward others should be stressed rather than ruthless competition.

Modern medicine has largely disregarded Hippocrates' simple method of treating illness by regimen (i.e., fasting, eating proper food, breathing fresh air, and resting and relaxing). Disease is the urgent attempt of the body to regain its normal state of health. This is called *vis medicatrix naturae*—the healing power of nature that cures from within. It is not easy for us to accept the theory that illness is the result of toxemia from inside our own bodies. It is more pleasant for us to accept Pasteur's theory that disease is caused by organisms from outside the body. It is one thing to wonder "Why did this have to happen to me?" and quite another to assume responsibility for one's own health.

Thus if you are sick, your pain, misery, and illness result from your wrong lifestyle (including dietary mistakes and the misuse or use of drugs). A century ago Dr. Oliver Wendell Holmes wrote a famous and oft-quoted statement: "I firmly believe if the whole *materia medica* as now used could be sunk to the bottom of the sea, it would be all the better for mankind—and all the worse for the fishes."

If you are sick, you are suffering because you are filled with toxic wastes caused by foods containing artificial preservatives, flavorings, and colors, and by foods devoid of vitamins and minerals. If you do select wholesome, natural foods, watch how you prepare them—do you boil the nutrition out of them by overcooking? Do you add harmful condiments to them? Harmful drugs, negative attitudes, and unhealthy living habits enable poisons, which have stagnated in your blood, to impair the filters and eliminative organs. These toxins are the real cause of disease. It is only when we realize this that Pasteur's theory that disease is caused by germs becomes relevant. After your cells have been damaged by toxic wastes, it is easy for bacteria to attack and devour the weakened, injured, and dead cells.

More and more people are becoming alarmed by the increased prevalence of major diseases despite a health industry estimated to spend around $150 billion per year. Greater numbers of people are becoming aware that true health care means preventing illnesses and maintaining optimum health by accepting individual responsibility. Courageous and often unorthodox physicians who eschew the tradition of attacking disease symptoms while ignoring causes are ushering in an age of new hope in the struggle for human health and happiness. All over America, programs have begun which focus on evaluating individual lifestyles and on ways of encouraging personal self-improvement for patients. Computerized evaluations contrast living habits with susceptibility to diseases, which is used at the Center for Disease Control in Atlanta.

The Atlanta program (sponsored by the United States Public Health Service), and others like it represent a monumental step away from the morass of medical treatment toward health care and disease prevention. In a democratic fashion, such programs make available the truth about a person's health and offer help to those who choose to take positive action. In the Atlanta program, over 1,400 federal employees fed information about their lives into a computer, an experiment which revealed their chances of living or dying during the next decade depending on whether those employees undertook corrective measures. Programs were offered that were designed to help the employees help themselves—programs to stop smoking, drink less, lose weight, change driving habits, reduce stress, improve nutrition, and increase physical exercise.

According to the director of the Atlanta program, H. G. Ogden, the "health hazard appraisal" has led to a response "far exceeding our expectations and the capacity of our facilities." Follow-ups and similar programs in Tucson and Duluth indicate that after eighteen months, employees involved in the project persist in their changed lifestyles.

Obviously, great gains in public health will become apparent when school curricula incorporate this wholistic methodology. If *all* our children were afforded knowledge, training, and guidance for healthy living, we would move beyond much of our self-made misery. Tennyson expressed this vision:

> Self-reference, self-knowledge, self-control,
> These three alone lead life to sovereign power.

For a vivid demonstration of the benefits of wholistic health care, it is useful to contrast that philosophy and practice with conventional medical treatment, as in the following chart.

Conventional Medical Treatment	Wholistic Health Care
*Focuses on treating symptoms	*Sees symptoms as a sign of imbalance in the whole organism
*Relies on drugs and surgery	*Avoids drugs and surgery in most instances
*Doctor-centered; he or she will promote health	*Person-centered: patient becomes responsible to avoid illness and build his or her health
*Sees the way to healing by attacking the disease in the tradition of Pasteur	*Sees the way to healing by strengthening the natural creative powers within—physical, emotional, mental, and spiritual—in the tradition of Hippocrates
*Tendency to ignore the nutrition and lifestyle of the person	*Stresses the relationship of nutrition and life habits to well-being
*Concerned with the physical aspects of health	*Concerned with all interrelated aspects of the whole person
*Frequent unawareness of harmful practices leading to iatrogenic (physician-caused) disease	*Deep respect for the inner healing power and the Hippocratic pledge to "first do no harm"
*Stresses treating illness	*Stresses the person's potential for greater health and happiness

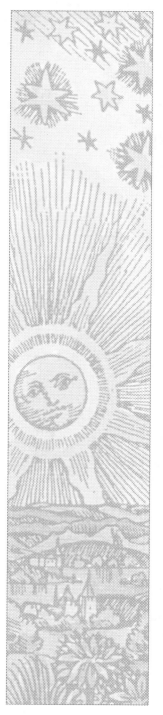

TWO

Food Can Be Your Medicine

When Not to Eat

Since elimination is so crucial to the life of our trillions of cells and to the body itself, there are times when we should abstain from food. Processing the fuel we put into our bodies and converting these substances into our blood, brain, muscle, bone, and organ cells is a monumental and energy-consuming task. Patients who are damaged by toxins from wrong foods and medications benefit from a fast of several days on vegetable broth along with bed rest. This allows "the doctor within us," to use Dr. Albert Schweitzer's phrase, to direct more energy to the work of elimination, cleansing, and healing. Dr. Alexis Carrel, the French Nobel prize-winning scientist, kept the cells of a chicken heart alive for almost thirty years by constantly removing the wastes of cell metabolism.

Animals have instinctive wisdom when it comes to abstaining from food, which most human beings have unfortunately forgotten. Instead we listen to that well-meaning inner parental record which says, "You'd better eat something anyway." But when animals are sick, upset, or wounded they know enough to fast and rest and only resume eating when they are well and their appetite returns. The true meaning of the saying "Feed a cold and starve a fever" is, "Feed a cold and you will have to starve a fever." A cold is not a disease; it is a healing action of the body in its attempt to eliminate toxins in one's system. So abstaining from food and all liquids (except pure water) and resting is the best way to help your body regain its health. Of course, with proper living and healthy nutrition one does not "catch" colds; the term *catch* implies that they come from outside. For myself and former patients on this wholistic way of living, a cold may occur once in many years, or not at all.

Eating when upset by anger, grief, or anxiety is also unwise. It is better to handle these feelings through some of the release exercises suggested in Chapter 8 of this book, and wait until you can feel relaxed and can draw a free breath before eating. With our system geared for emergency fight or flight, even the most wholesome food will not be properly digested under stress. Obese individuals often eat compulsively when they are in a state of tension or rage, hate themselves for being fat, and become caught in this vicious circle. Periods of mourning can also be a normal and necessary experience that should not be swallowed down with food. Experiencing our feelings, including the painful ones, can lead to catharsis, self-understanding, and growth. Similarly, physical pain is a sign that should lead us to find the cause and deal with it constructively, rather than deaden the pain with food or drugs.

Animals also have an instinctual ability, in their natural habitat, to choose the proper foods for their biological makeup. Those closest to humans physiologically—the primates—build healthy bodies and great strength on mother's milk, and on fruits and vegetation and little animal protein, if any, after they have been weaned. The healthiest people of the world (such as the Hunzas of Asia, the people of Vilcabamba in Ecuador, and the people of the Balkans) live far longer and healthier lives than we do in affluent, industrialized societies. The degenerative diseases which plague us (e.g., cancer, heart disease, circulatory and alimentary illnesses, arthritis, and diabetes) are almost unheard of in these societies. Although stress, pollution, and lack of physical exercise are negative components of industrialization that contribute to ill health, we have much to learn about nutrition from animals and people who live in accord with the laws of nature.

Jane—A Case of Digging One's Grave with One's Teeth

Jane is a perfect example of the disastrous effects of eating refined and unnatural foods. She had spent years and a fortune on psychiatrists and psychoanalysts, seeking a cure for her panic and anxiety states, mood swings, fatigue, weakness, addictive tendencies, headaches, and depression. The psychiatric drugs made her feel like a zombie; the analysis made her more and more turned in and preoccupied with herself.

Syntonics examines the whole lifestyle of the person, so when Jane came to me as a last resort (not an uncommon occurrence), I explored her dietary habits. She had many cups of coffee a day with two spoons of sugar, along with doughnuts and other white flour pastries to "pick up my energy." I sensed a serious threat to her health and referred her to my wholistic colleague, Dr. Azim Etemadi, for a glucose tolerance test. Sure enough, she was "off the graph" for hypoglycemia (i.e., low blood sugar), which accounted for a large part of her symptoms. Her other doctors had wrongly assumed that all her problems were psychological.

What causes hypoglycemia, a serious disturbance afflicting perhaps 20 percent of the U.S. population and linked to crime, truancy, divorce, violence, accidents, and depression?[1] Sugar and white flour introduce substances into the body that are devoid of the vitamins and minerals necessary for their digestion and assimilation. This triggers the pancreas to produce an excessive amount of insulin and pushes the sugar level below normal. The body responds to this "state of emergency" and produces adrenaline to mobilize the system. A vicious circle occurs when the person repeats the same destructive behavior to get another "pick-up"; the scenario is often worsened by an accompanying cigarette habit.

The cure is simple: a healthy diet of whole grains, raw and steamed vegetables, low-fat cottage cheese with omega 3 flax oil, unsalted nuts and seeds, (but no dates or raisins), and (for nonvegetarians) fish, poultry, and seafood. Restorative vitamin and mineral supplements are also indicated. Ideally, intramuscular supplementation by a wholistic, nutritionally oriented physician (such as Drs. Azim Etemadi, Robert Wallis, and Robert Atkins in New York City) will bring the system back to harmony more effectively. This disturbance is a forerunner of a major dis-

---

[1] Marilyn Light, "A Quick Look At Hypoglycemia," International Homeopathic Alliance Ltd., New York, N.Y., 1985.

ease—diabetes—which occurs when the insulin factory is depleted. Again, as Syntonics never tires of stressing, prevention of illness through healthy eating, breathing, exercising, thinking, feeling, and being is the bottom line.

Happily once Jane's physical health was restored she had the energy to resolve her personal problems and achieve emotional security, self-esteem, peace of mind, and spiritual serenity.

Are You Eating Like a Gorilla or a Tiger?

Increasing numbers of health and nutritional experts agree that Americans consume far too much animal fat in their diet. These saturated fats play a major part in heart disease (which takes a million lives prematurely per year) in the U.S.; high blood pressure (which affects approximately thirty million people); and cancer (which has increased about 250 percent in the last several decades).

The Protein Myth

Most of us have been led to believe that protein is the essence of a healthy diet and that without slabs of meat, and milk, cheese, and eggs every day, we would curl up and fade away. These high fat foods have status as the center of a meal, are more expensive than healthy whole grains, beans and vegetables, and have an aura of success about them. And yet they are part of the current American diet, which is helping to keep our hospitals full, our disease rates increasing, and our undertakers overworked.

What is protein? It is a group of common chemical substances called amino acids. These are arranged in strings, like beads, to form protein. There are twenty-two amino

acids that comprise the proteins which are known at the
present time. Most nutritionists say that eight of these,
called essential amino acids, are the ones our bodies are not
able to manufacture. Unfortunately, we have been led to
believe that only by eating animal flesh can we obtain these
necessary amino acids. If this were so, billions of vegetari-
ans in the world (who, incidentally, are free from many of
our killer diseases) could not possibly survive, much less
live longer and more vigorous lives than we.

Nor does meat contain more protein than certain other
foods. Cheese, sunflower seeds, and some nuts contain
higher concentrations of protein than meat. In fact, all foods
contains some protein, including fruits and vegetables; obviously, the largest and strongest animals in the world build
their bodies from the protein in vegetable matter. This is not
too surprising when we consider that the percentage of protein in mother's milk is designed to enable the infant to *double* its weight in the first few months of life. What would you
guess this percentage to be? Most people I ask, including
nutritionists and physicians, suggest a figure of 10 to 50 percent. However, the answer is 2 percent, which is close to the
amount of protein found in fruits and vegetables. This gives
us another clue to the prevalence of degenerative diseases in
affluent countries. Too much of anything can be bad and out
of balance with nature. The average person needs only
about thirty-five or forty grams—a bit over an ounce—of
protein per day.[2] Excessive amounts can become toxic and
strain the kidneys and other organs of elimination.

Is meat essential in your diet to ensure adequate protein
intake? Obviously not. The healthiest longest lived people

---

[1] *Canadian Bulletin on Nutrition—Dietary Standard for Canada,* 1964.

of the world: the Hunzas, the Abkhasians, and the people of Vilcabamba, thrive with little or no meat. The Seventh-Day Adventists in America who follow their vegetarian teaching are known to be much healthier and longer-lived than the average American stuffed with excess meat and animal products. Another important consideration in the championing of less meat consumption is that more and more animals and chickens bred for food consumption contain pesticides and carcinogenic hormones that are injected to fatten them up. You can derive all the necessary vitamins and minerals you need from whole and natural grains, sprouts, vegetables, fruits, seeds, and nuts—for far less money than the cost of processed foods and meat. An additional bonus is that you will avoid contributing to the $150 billion or more spent annually on our gigantic (and often unnecessary) "health" industry, drugs and surgery.

Robert C. Atkins, M.D., whose complementary approach uses proper nutrition and individualized supplementation to overcome illness by creating health, states that "a quarter of a million heart bypasses are done yearly (at a cost of $50,000-$100,000 apiece) when prestigious studies show that more than half are inappropriate."[3]

George Bernard Shaw supposedly once exclaimed, "I refuse to make my stomach the burial ground for a dead pig." It is purely myth that meat eaters are better fed than those, like myself, who choose seafood and occasionally fowl. For the high content of fat in meat and other animal products not only clogs up the body's blood vessels, but leads to obesity. There is no obesity or heart disease among the vegetarian Bantu of Africa!

---

[3] Dr. Atkins Health-Revelations—Nov. 1993—Vol. I, No. 9 p. 1.

The Importance of a High-Fiber Diet

Meat also lacks another element of paramount importance in human nutrition: fiber. Fiber is the solid material in whole grains, vegetables, and fruits (in their natural or nearly raw state) which passes through the body virtually undigested with a cleansing effect.

Fiber is essential in the process of elimination, which enables us to get rid of the waste products that otherwise accumulate in our cells, tissues and organs. Dr. Ernst Wynder, a physician who heads the American Health Foundation, states:

> Most of the major chronic diseases that we suffer from today are totally man-made. To die of cancer or arteriosclerosis is not an inevitable consequence of aging. The only true cause of death should be when each person's individual genetic time clock runs out.

What has this to do with meat eating and fiber in our food? Dr. Wynder links the "same type of diet" with both cancer and heart disease, namely a diet in which much animal food and little fiber is present. He further states:

> Currently high rates of colon cancer can be directly linked to a high bile-acid content in a person's stool. The average person in the United States has an extremely high level of bile-acid in their stools. When patients were placed on a meat free diet, within four weeks their bile acid levels dropped significantly.[4]

---

[4]E.L. Wynder, "Strategies Toward the Primary Prevention of Cancer." *Archives of Surgery*, Volume 125, p. 163-169.

Additionally, Dr. Wynder emphasizes that there occurs a far lower rate of breast cancer among vegetarian women who maintain a low fat and high fiber diet. These women produce 40% less prolactin, a substance linked with breast cancer.[5]

Healing Arthritis

It is estimated that 25,000,000 Americans suffer from joint problems called osteoarthritis (degenerative joint disease). Several factors are suspect: food allergies, vitamin and mineral deficiencies, poor diet, and bowel toxins. It is common knowledge that drugs may ease the pain but fail to deal with the causes, and they may produce severe side-effects, called iatrogenic disease. Here is how you can help yourself.

1. Remember that a low-fat (10 percent) diet of whole grains, fruits, vegetables, except night shades (peppers, tomatoes, eggplant and potatoes) fiber, and seafood has proven itself in many societies that are relatively free of this disease.
2. Check yourself for food allergies using the methods described in Chapter 4.
3. Make sure you are taking a natural-source vitamin and mineral supplement.[6]
4. Supplement your high-fiber diet with psyllium husks powder, taken morning and night in juice or water for a clean colon.

---

[5] E.L. Wynder, "Cancer Prevention: Optimizing Lifestyles With Special Reference to Nutritional Carcinogens," *Journal of The National Cancer Institute,* Monograph, Vol. i2 pp. 87-91.

[6] I recommend Basic Formula #1 from The Atkins Center for Complementary Medicine, 152 E. 56 St, New York, N.Y. 10022.

5. If necessary, see a nutritional doctor (who might find you to be deficient in zinc, selenium, and manganese, which is often the case in arthritic patients).

I also recommend taking six fish oil and primrose capsules each day. Seven herbs like comfrey, devil's claw, and parsley tea can help with hot castor oil packs.

In the June 1993 issue of his exciting and trail-blazing newsletter *Health and Healing,* Dr. Julian Whitaker warns of the dangers of the drugs commonly used for arthritis, such as aspirin, Motrin, Naprosyn, Feldene, etc.[7] He maintains that these nonsteroidal, antiinflammatory drugs (NSAIDS) not only cause intestinal bleeding in close to 25,000 people a year but, even worse, "block the body's ability to produce cartilage and actually cause cartilage destruction. . . . Indocin is a powerful and very dangerous NSAID. In Norway, a group of patients taking Indocin were found to have far more rapid destruction of the hip than the group not taking Indocin."

The good news is that there is a natural substance, called glucosamine, which is necessary for the body in healing and repairing joint surfaces. Dr. Whitaker eliminates all NSAIDS with his patients, over a one- or two-week period, and then has the patient use four capsules of glucosamine sulfate for at least a six-week period. (Call Enzymatic Therapy, in Green Bay, Wisconsin, at 414-469-1313 for health food stores in your area that carry it. It comes in 500-mg capsules and costs about $20 for sixty capsules.) Along with this and a healthy, low-fat diet and supplementary vitamins and minerals, Dr. Whitaker also recommends two

---

[7] Dr. Julian Whitaker, *Health and Healing.* June 1993, p. 4, Phillips Publishing, Inc.

teaspoons daily of spray-dried barley grass juice—Barley green, Green Magma, or Kyo-green.

If you are under a doctor's care, discuss this break-through with him or her. If your doctor is not open to new and better approaches, find a nutritional physician who is. (See listings after Appendix.)

Recently I saw an interview on T.V. with the actor James Coburn who spoke of his struggle with arthritis. He went on a fifteen day fast and had a number of colonics (a special method of cleansing one's colon), both of which greatly helped his body cleanse itself and also relieved the pain in body joints. A fast of pure water, or vegetable broth is also recommended by many wholistic doctors, perhaps one day every two weeks as a general aid to health and longevity. For longer fasts, if you have any particular health problems, be receptive to the guidance of a nutritional physician.

The Secret of Losing Weight Without Yo-Yo Diets

I agree with my colleague Julian Whitaker, M.D., that there is only one weight loss approach that really works without doing harm. It is simple! The natural, traditional, whole, low-fat foods of many cultures—our prudent Syntonic way of eating—along with physical activity natu-rally kept people in shape. The long-lived people of Hunza, near Tibet, for example, were vital and slim, except for their king (who gave banquets, traveled, and lived the "rich" life full of meats, dairy, and refined foods). He was the only fat one in group photos, and he was destined for a much shorter life—the bigger the waistline, the shorter the lifeline.

The 30 percent fat diet recommended by the American Heart Association is inadequate to eliminate excess weight, high cholesterol, and the risk of diabetes. The low fat approach does amazing things on all four levels of the person, and it leads to renewed enthusiasm and vital spirituality. Take the following steps for a month, and see for yourself.

12 Steps in a Sound Weight Loss Program

1. Enjoy whole grains, vegetables, salads, beans, legumes, and (if desired) occasional seafood or skinless poultry. Stress sprouted and raw foods (See appendix VI).
2. Think low protein and high fiber.
3. Avoid packaged and processed foods, dairy, margarine, and hydrogenated fats and oils—except olive, canola, and flaxseed (omega 3 oil), all of which are ideal with apple cider vinegar for salad dressing.
4. After a while on the low-fat regime, you will no longer desire greasy, rich, fatty foods. Avoid all sugars, simple carbohydrates, milk (lactose), and fruit juices.
5. You will lose weight without feeling hungry because of eating so little fat, but ample bulk and fiber. Avoid MSG, corn syrup, flour, pickling, nitrites and all preservatives.
6. Emphasize whole grain or artichoke pastas; cereals without sugar, salt, or fat; nonfat dairy products; tofu and soy soups.
7. Make sure you exercise regularly (the equivalent of a half-hour walk five times a week). You *must* burn fat and speed up your metabolism.

8. To reduce stress (which may lead to overeating), use the methods outlined in chapters 7 and 8 to improve your well-being.

9. With less fat and more fiber, your body will also be cleaner, your energy level will be increased, your clearer blood will flow more easily through your capillaries, your brain will get more oxygen, the fatty plaques in your arteries will shrink, you will feel more calm and energetic, and you will probably live a longer, happier, and fuller life free of the killer diseases of "civilization" if you also care for your emotions, mind and Spirit.

10. Take psyllium powder every day to avoid self-poisoning from your colon. Dr. James F. Balch (op. cit. p. 32) lists hemorrhoids, varicose veins, obesity, indigestion, diverticulitis, appendicitis, hernia, and bowel cancer as some of the ailments arising from a clogged colon. There is truth in the old saying: "death begins in the colon."

11. Here's something to write home about; a new fat called a medium chain triglyceride (MCT) that acts more like a carbohydrate than a fat. Instead of weight gain, it causes weight loss. In contrast, the long chain (LCTs) found in butter, meat, cheese, and coconut oil, according to Dr. Julian Whitaker, not only put on weight, but "are associated with heart disease and cancer." He goes on to note that in one study the amount of calories burned after six hours on a meal containing MCTs was almost twice as high as after a meal containing LCTs.

This should encourage you! He mentions a 42-year-old male, already on a low-fat and exercise regimen, who started using MCTs as a spread on whole grain bread and as a salad oil. In four months he lost 30 pounds.

Health food stores carry MCT oil products. Twin Labs (MCT Fuel) is about $11 for a 16 oz. bottle. The actual amount of MCTs is four grams per tablespoon. Dr. Whitaker suggests taking one or two spoons per day and cautions that diabetics should be under a doctor's care if they use them.[8]

12. As a counterpart to your healthy green tea, there is also a tea containing ephedra, a substance that also helps to shed weight. It can be ordered through Vitamin Research Products; 800-877-2447. With certain medical conditions this is not advised, so ask when you call (they are listed on the label). It is called thermagen herbal tea.

Fiber for Disease Prevention

Perhaps the most famous name in the fantastic story of fiber relating to disease prevention is that of Denis Burkitt, an English medical anthropologist. Dr. Burkitt is a physician who has a deep knowledge of nutrition (unlike most doctors, who are trained only to treat symptoms with drugs and surgery). Burkitt indicates that although statistically the average human lifespan has increased,

in actuality the life expectancy of a person who reaches the age of 45 has not changed since the late 1800s. In other words, the population of 100 years ago lost many of its

---

[8]J. Whitaker, *Health and Healing*, July 1993, Vol. 3, No. 7.

members to infectious diseases early in life. Presently we have eliminated most deaths due to infectious disease but modern medicine has in no way affected death due to degenerative disease (cancer, heart disease, etc.). In fact these diseases have been on the increase.[9]

Dr. Burkitt's explanation for this situation has to do with nutrition and that simple, down-to-earth substance called fiber. Over the last ninety years, technological "progress" enabled us to mill and refine rice and grains. The natural diet of whole grains on which human beings have thrived throughout their evolution, has been destroyed. The plague of heart disease, cancer, and diabetes has burgeoned along with white flour, white rice and white sugar. In our ambition to control nature, we have violated the natural laws of nutrition. One of my favorite quotations is from the philosopher Francis Bacon: "Man can only conquer Nature by obeying her!"

"One of the key factors," proclaims Dr. Burkitt, "has been the elimination of fiber from our diets. This dietary fiber, most available in the form of unrefined cooked grains, appears to be the key in preventing a myriad of diseases." This may sound like a glib promise of a magical remedy, but it derives from one of the leading health experts of modern years. Some of the diseases Burkitt cites as examples improved or prevented by the incorporation of a high-fiber diet are diabetes, cancer of the colon, appendicitis, hiatal hernia, varicose veins, and diverticular disease. No wonder Syntonics stresses a high-fiber diet!

The work of Burkitt and other researchers was done with natives in Africa. Although Africans have some of the

[9]Life Span, Vol. 3, No. 2.

infectious diseases associated with poor sanitation, they are nonetheless free from those diseases that are connected with an intake of heavy animal food and low fiber. Heart disease is a rarity among these people since fiber, whole grains, and vegetables are their native diet. Among the Bantus, for example, whose diet contains about 10 percent fat (the American diet contains about 40 percent fat), heart disease is almost unknown! Autopsies performed on Europeans living in Africa but consuming little fiber and much meat revealed that 10 percent of this group of twenty-two people, including a fifteen-year-old boy, had severe artery damage.[10]

Natives of New Guinea, whose high-fiber, natural food, vegetarian diet contains about 10 percent fat and 7 percent protein, showed only one case of heart disease in 600 cases. They also demonstrated no rise in blood pressure with age; in fact, their diastolic pressure dropped about 10 mm when they reached their sixties.[11]

Another group of people in Vilcabamba, Ecuador, who live to the age of one hundred or more, were found to be free of clogged arteries and heart disease. These Ecuadorians subsist on a high-fiber, and low-fat diet of complex (unrefined) carbohydrates—corn, beans, vegetables, fruits, brown rice—with a small portion of meat about once a week.[12]

Thus, the right fuel for that miraculous self-healing organism, your body, is essential for its repair and maintenance. The diet endorsed by Syntonics prevents or cures gallstones, which are crystals of cholesterol that form in the

---

[10]J. B. Hannah, *Central African Journal of Medicine,* Vol. 4, pp. 1-5, 1958.

[11]A.M. Whyte, *Aust. Ann. Med.,* Vol. 7, pp. 36, 47, 1958.

[12]A. Leaf, "Hard Labor, Low Cholesterol Linked to Unusual Longevity," *Medical Tribune,* June 1971.

gallbladder and may block the secretion of bile into the small intestine. Such gallstones are aggravated by a wrong diet and lack of fiber.[13] Similarly, James Balch, M.D., points to bad diet as a cause of gout, a condition resulting from the accumulation of too much uric acid in the body from excessive meat eating. He recommends two weeks of raw fruits and vegetables.[14]

Even ulcers seem to have a correlation with the foods we select, in addition to stress and anxiety. Researchers conducting a study in England gave a group of subjects meals of white bread and, at different times, meals of whole wheat bread.[15] The rate at which food left the subjects' stomachs were then measured. When fiber-depleted white bread was eaten, the liquid contents of the stomach, including stomach acid, passed on to the small intestine much more rapidly than after the subjects had eaten whole wheat bread. The duodenum, the first part of the small intestine, is a common location for an ulcer to occur. Happily, since we create these diseases ourselves, with knowledge and discipline we can become our own doctors working with the healing intelligence within to prevent or heal these self-made sicknesses.

The fast pace of modern life parallels our fast pace of eating quick and deadly junk foods. Nutrients are absorbed more quickly into our blood stream, unnaturally so. But we cannot fool the natural order of life. Such a fast pace, taking shortcuts by means of fast foods, is very undesirable for our digestive function.

---

[13] *Lancet*, August 12, 1978.

[14] Op. cit. p. 32.

[15] *Lancet*, October 1, 1977.

On the subject of fruit and fruit juice, which do you think could be damaging in the long run to your body? Researchers discovered that after drinking a quantity of apple juice, insulin levels rose much higher than after having a meal of apples! This too-sudden intake of sugar from the juice triggered a larger amount of insulin than normal to regulate the blood sugar level, which in turn created a below normal drop in the body's blood sugar level. This insidious condition is called hypoglycemia, or hyper (too much) insulinism. The fiber from whole apples, on the contrary, combined with the slower chewing and swallowing process, avoids that jolt to the insulin factory, the pancreas. Too many shocks in this manner over the years leads to another man-made potentially fatal illness, diabetes.[16]

Fiber is essential to the proper functioning of the colon. Those who eat too much meat and fat and refined carbohydrates find they even produce unnatural stools. The healthy fibrous ones are larger and absorb more fluids. Healthy stools aid in diluting poisons that may cause cancer, and prevent these toxins from becoming reabsorbed by the body in a process of self-intoxication. Larger, protective stools pass more quickly through the body facilitating the peristaltic action of the muscles, and avoid pressure in the bowel that may create little pouches or diverticulosis. A study by Drs. Brodribb and Humphreys at the Royal Berkshire Hospital in Reading, England, found that an ounce of wheat bran daily, for six months, led to 60 percent of gout symptoms abolished, and 28 percent of them relieved.[17]

Additional problems that may arise from straining to

---

[16] *Lancet*, October 1, 1977.

[17] *British Medical Journal*, February 21, 1976.

eliminate fiberless stools from the body are (1) hiatal hernia (a stomach pouch protruding through the diaphragm), (2) varicose veins (pushing blood back through the veins of the legs), and (3) distension of the veins of the rectum (hemorrhoids). Moreover, a recent study that explored the relationship between diet and heart disease among 337 subjects over a period of ten years demonstrated that those subjects with the highest cereal fiber intake had the lowest rate of heart disease. [18]

Clearly, fiber-rich foods grown without chemicals are as healthful to eat as fractured foods such as white sugar, white rice, and white flour are detrimental to health. [19]

Refined Foods and Their Dangers

Adulterated foods such as those mentioned earlier are known as refined foods. One must not assume that they are pure and respectable, as that term might suggest. All of the diseases cited previously are connected with the consumption of sugar, which may be the most destructive culprit of all. John Yudkin, M.D., an eminent British nutritionist, relates sugar intake to "an increase in cholesterol, triglycerides, enlarged liver, damaged kidneys, impaired glucose tolerance, and insulin insensitivity". [20]

A common evil of white sugar is its tendency to increase dental problems and tooth decay. However, workers in cane

---

[18] For extra fiber, two spoonsful of miller's bran may be taken in water before each meal, or with soups and other foods.

[19] The Feingold Diet has shown the importance of eliminating all candies, chemical additives and dyestuffs from the food intake of hyperactive children, rather than deadening them with drugs and medications.

[20] *New Dynamics of Preventive Medicine*, Vol. 3, p. 68, 1975.

fields, who chew the cane itself and ingest the minerals, enzymes, vitamins, and fiber of the cane, have had little problem with cavities and dental decay. This is another example of how eating a whole food in its natural state reflects harmonious assimilation of the cosmic plan.

Dr. Yudkin correlates the epidemic of heart disease with the fact that the intake of white sugar in America has risen about eight times since 1900 and the average American now consumes well over 100 pounds of sugar per year. Sugar is used as a cheap filler in everything from bread and cereal to ketchup and frankfurters, so unless you read labels and are nutritionally aware, you may be suffering sugar damage without realizing it.

Sugar has also been connected to epidemics of both colon cancer and rectal cancer. There is evidence that sugar alters the dominant type of bacteria residing in the colon and subsequently acts as a carcinogen.[21] Not only is sugar devoid of vitamins, minerals, and enzymes, but it has *no fiber*, a trait which interferes with our elimination system and encourages the destructive powers of harmful bacteria.

Sugar — The White Plague

Sugar and its cousins, fiberless white flour and white rice, also disturb the blood sugar level of the body. A jolt of sugar into the system sends the sugar level of the blood up too quickly (as does a cigarette, coffee, or even a large glass of fruit juice), and forces the body to emit insulin to restore a normal sugar balance. The excessive sugar stimulus then results in an excessive amount of insulin, which results in a "low" after the "high." Low blood sugar, or hypoglycemia, is

---

[21] M. J. Hill et al., *Lancet*, Vol. 1, pp. 95-99.

recognized as a growing illness by the *Journal of the American Medical Association.*[22] In an article published in that journal, Dr. S. H. Newmark writes that

> in cases of severe, chronic hypoglycemia, central nervous system function is profoundly altered, and I have seen patients display symptoms ranging from headache, change in affect (emotions), anorexia (lack of appetite), irritability, lethargy, and even psychotic behavior or frank coma.

Likewise, Syntonics stresses the connection between poor diet (sugar, caffeine, nicotine, white flour, pastries, etc.) and emotional disturbances.

In my wholistic method of therapy, I have found it important to review the diet of my patients which is often neglected by psychotherapists. It is possible to get the "sugar blues" and to enter anxiety states because of indulging in coffee breaks several times a day, imbibing sugared coffee and snacking on sweets and sugar-loaded pastries made of white flour; and then engorging in meals high in meat and fat content. The accumulated use of sugar over a period of time can finally exhaust the insulin factory in your pancreas resulting in *diabetes mellitus*, or sugar diabetes. Until the peoples of Greenland, India, Yemen, New Guinea, Polynesia, and Trinidad were introduced to sugar by other nations, they were free of diabetic diseases. (Again, sugar diabetes is another human-made condition that can be prevented through correct nourishment.) Further, during World Wars I and II, when the "luxuries" of white sugar and white flour were unavailable, both the incidence of diabetes, heart disease, and the death rate among civilians

---

[22] "Hyperglycemia and Hypoglycemia Crises," Vol. 231, No. 2, 1975.

declined appreciably. Treatment of diabetes by means of diet and exercise prescribed by wholistic doctors has often mitigated or ended the need for insulin injections.

Cleaves Bennett, M.D., Medical Director of the Longevity Center in Santa Monica, California, illustrates the effect of diet in producing diabetes as seen in the population of the small island of Naru in the South Pacific. When the dietary intake took a radical shift from simple island foods to over-refined, high-fat Western foods, almost the entire adult population became clinically classified as diabetic and obese. This occurred over a roughly two-year period. Bennett reports that the program at the Center, by reducing caloric fat and sugar intake and increasing physical activity, resulted in "a marked improvement in glucose utilization and a reduction in the need for insulin or oral agents." [23]

Refined sugar and grains also rob your body of B vitamins, which are necessary for digestion and metabolism. Whole foods provide an appropriate amount of such vitamins. When the average American diet depletes them, metabolism is incomplete. Lactic acid, instead of being converted to glycogen (usable energy), begins to circulate in the blood stream, inducing fatigue, poor memory, slow thinking, irritability, and disturbed and anxious emotional states. The combination of low blood sugar and the depletion of the B vitamins has vast implications not only for physical health, but also for social health and human behavior. It has been observed that the symptoms associated with low blood sugar are so similar to the emotional, mental, and behavioral symptoms of severe psychogenic or neurotic ill-

---

[23] *Life Span,* Vol. 3, No. 2.

READER/CUSTOMER CARE SURVEY

If you are enjoying this book, please help us serve you better and meet your changing needs by taking a few minutes to complete this survey. Please fold it & drop it in the mail. **As a thank you, we will send you a gift.**

Name: _____

Address: _____

_____

Tel. # _____

(1) Gender: 1) ____ Female 2) ____ Male

(2) Age:
1)____ 18-25   4)____ 46-55
2)____ 26-35   5)____ 56-65
3)____ 36-45   6)____ 65+

(3) Marital status:

1)____ Married 3)____ Single 5)____ Widowed
2)____ Divorced 4)____ Partner

(4) Is this book:
1)____ Purchased for self?
2)____ Purchased for others?
3)____ Received as gift?

(5) How did you find out about this book?

1)____ Catalog 2)____ Store Display
Newspaper
3)____ Best Seller List
4)____ Article/Book Review
5)____ Advertisement
Magazine
6)____ Feature Article
7)____ Book Review
8)____ Advertisement
9)____ Word of Mouth
A)____ T.V./Talk Show (Specify) _____
B)____ Radio/Talk Show (Specify) _____
C)____ Professional Referral _____
D)____ Other (Specify) _____

(6) What subject areas do you enjoy reading most? (Rank in order of enjoyment)

1)____ Women's Issues/   5)____ New Age/
Relationships   Altern. Healing
2)____ Business Self Help   6)____ Aging
3)____ Soul/Spirituality/   7)____ Parenting
Inspiration   8)____ Diet/Nutrition/
4)____ Recovery   Exercise/Health

(14) What do you look for when choosing a personal growth book?
(Rank in order of importance)

1)____ Subject   3)____ Author
2)____ Title   4)____ Price
Cover Design   5)____ In Store Location

(19) When do you buy books?
(Rank in order of importance)

1)____ Christmas
2)____ Valentine's Day
3)____ Birthday
4)____ Mother's Day
5)____ Other (Specify _____

(23) Where do you buy your books?
(Rank in order of frequency of purchases)

1)____ Bookstore   6)____ Gift Store
2)____ Price Club   7)____ Book Club
3)____ Department Store   8)____ Mail Order
4)____ Supermarket/   9)____ T.V. Shopping
Drug Store   A)____ Airport
5)____ Health Food Store

Which book are you currently reading? _____

Additional comments you would like to make to help us serve you better.

_____

_____

Thank You !!

NO POSTAGE
NECESSARY
IF MAILED
IN THE
UNITED STATES

BUSINESS REPLY MAIL

FIRST CLASS MAIL PERMIT NO 45 DEERFIELD BEACH, FL

POSTAGE WILL BE PAID BY ADDRESSEE

HEALTH COMMUNICATIONS
3201 SW 15TH STREET
DEERFIELD BEACH, FL 33442-9875

nesses that unaware doctors often treat one mistakenly for the other.[24]

In writing about the effect of refined carbohydrates and white sugar, Adelle Davis comments with prophetic insight into our own violent society, including among youth, 40 years later:

> the resulting irritability, nervous tension and mental depression are such that a person can easily go berserk. If hatred, bitterness and resentments are harbored and a temporary psychological upset causes a person to go on a candy binge . . . the stage is set . . . [and] violence and quarreling can occur for which there may be no forgiving. Add a few guns, gas jets, or razor blades, and you have the stuff murders and suicides are made of. The American diet has become dangerous in more ways than one.[25]

The Magic of Syntonic Eating

What are the right foods to eat? The basic principle is to eat foods in their natural state, with nothing taken from them and nothing added to them. They must also be appropriate to the human constitution. Since humans are biologically similar to the primates (not the carnivores), food should be derived mainly from the vegetable kingdom. Every mineral, vitamin, enzyme, and every known and unknown substance you need is contained in natural foods raised naturally and allowed to remain so. (The ideal is to have your own organic garden. However, health stores and markets often offer natural produce.) The new wholistic

---

[24] E. M. Abrahamson, M.D., *Body, Mind and Sugar,* Henry Holt and Co., N.Y., 1951.

[25] *Let's Eat Right to Keep Fit,* Adelle Davis, New American Library, 1954.

way of living, which avoids medications, is training doctors of health to practice the Hippocratic philosophy: "Let your food be your medicine."

The conventional American diet, which enables countless Americans to "dig their graves with their teeth," derives about 40 percent of its calories from fat, about 20 percent from protein, and about 40 percent from carbohydrates (the latter mostly refined carbohydrates). The Syntonic diet which I recommend to my patients is radically different in both quantity and quality.

This prudent diet is high on those wonder foods—whole brown rice and whole grains (wheat, oats, barley, millet, and corn)—organically raised in naturally enriched earth, free from chemical insecticides. Along with a variety of beans, peas, lentils, seasonal fruits, and fresh vegetables, eaten raw or lightly steamed, these complex (complete) carbohydrates comprise about 80 percent of the total calories of this high-energy nourishment. The balance is about 10 percent fats (olive, flax seed, and canola oil) and 10 percent protein, mostly from seafoods, fowl, and unsalted nuts and seeds.

This diet is also the traditional longevity diet of people all over the globe who live in four-season climates and who have not fallen prey to the typical "civilized" diet (huge quantities of dairy, meat, sugar, processed, low-fiber foods) that has inaugurated the scourge of degenerative, human-made illnesses.

On this Syntonic diet, breakfast might consist of

Raw fruits or fruit compote
  (no fruit if you are hypoglycemic)

Oats with fruit, sunflower seeds, pumpkin seeds, lecithin
   granules, and brewer's yeast (a rich source of the vital
   B vitamins)
Herb tea, whole grain toast, apple butter or sesame butter
   with a small amount of organic honey (if you don't have
   a problem with low blood sugar).
   (If in doubt get a glucose tolerance test.)

Lunch might consist of

A large salad with homemade dressing made with apple
   cider vinegar and omega 3 flax oil. (Along with fish oil,
   flax oil is the best source of essential fatty acids. These
   "good" fats and oils have been shown to reduce the
   development of high cholesterol, autoimmune diseases,
   and heart disease.) [26]
You may also have a cold beet soup or a hot vegetable or
   lentil or pea soup (depending on the season) and whole
   grain toast, sesame butter, and either herb tea or a coffee substitute.
A brown rice casserole with steamed vegetables (such as
   carrots, onions, and broccoli) with low-salt soy sauce, a
   small salad, and herb tea or a coffee substitute[fo]

Dinner might consist of

A whole grain casserole (brown rice, millet, bulghur
   wheat, or barley) with a variety of steamed vegetables,
   and a salad with a healthy dressing (see above).
   Nonvegetarians may add steamed fish or other seafood
   or skinless chicken.

---

[26] *Journal of the American Medical Assn.*, Feb. 1982.

A brown rice and mixed bean casserole, with steamed vegetables on the side, and a mixed salad (as above). Eat
enough so you have no room for desert. Rather finish
your meal with herb tea or a coffee substitute.

In addition, it's a good idea to drink bottled spring water
or filter your tap water.

Julian Whitaker, M.D., is one of my favorite wholistic
physicians and editor of the excellent monthly report
Health and Healing (Phillips Pub. Inc.). He suggests that as
a start you become a vegetarian for two days per week, eating only fruits, vegetables, and whole grains (including
whole grain pastas). Dr. Whitaker says, "Your kidneys will
love you for it, so will your bones. In fact, your whole body
will rejoice." At the same time you will be cutting out animal fat, which he says is a factor in heart disease, cancer,
and hypertension. You will probably lose weight, too.
Some of my patients have lost as much as a hundred
pounds in one year in this way (cutting way down on animal fat, sugar, and white flour desserts), but eating freely
of healthy foods plus exercising.

Another danger to your health is margarine, which is
composed of oil that is made solid (hydrogenated) by alter-
ing its molecular structure. Margarine (originally touted as
a no-cholesterol substitute for butter) is used in a wide
variety of cookies, crackers, and many other processed
foods, and it is now seen as a substance the body cannot
handle (this substance is called trans-fatty acid). In a study
presented at the 1993 American Heart Association meeting, Dr. Alberto Ascherio of Harvard University disclosed
his study of heart attack victims. Those whose diets were
highest in trans-fatty acids had 2.44 times the rate of heart
attacks as those who ate the lowest amount of trans-fatty

acids.) So use olive oil, flax oil, or a small amount of unsalted butter on your whole grain bread. Give your heart the break it deserves!

Some years ago, I worked with Long Island residents on this diet along with exercise and stress-reduction techniques. The results were as follows: significant weight loss in overweight clients, reduction of high blood pressure (for most, a cessation of the need for drugs), significant lowering of cholesterol levels and blood fat levels, and the elimination or lessening of the need for insulin in diabetics.[27]

A number of "new" wholistically oriented health experts are also enthusiastic about this 80-10-10 diet. Dr. James Anderson of the University of Kentucky says, "It's a magic diet—it could save a significant number of lives." Dr. Cleaves Bennett of UCLA eulogizes that "If Americans went on the 80-10-10 diet, we would just about not have hypertension, coronary heart disease or strokes, and very few complications of hardening of the arteries." Dr. Julian Whitaker, also director of the California Heart Treatment Center in San Clemente, California, observes, "This is the way much of the world eats which doesn't have the disease problems we have." A heart specialist, Dr. Paul Dudley White, quotes Leviticus 7:23 as a parallel to this way of eating: "Ye shall eat no manner of fat, of ox, or of sheep, or of goat."

---

[27] The New Horizon diet and the findings related to it were very similar to the results obtained at the Longevity Center in California and its Pritikin diet. However, at the New Horizon Center we also stressed the emotional and psychological aspects of well-being toward effective self-maintenance in the total Syntonic approach.

Dairy Products

Many health experts point out that the only milk appropriate for human beings is that perfect food for babies — mother's milk.[28] After weaning, people who thrive on natural, whole food throughout the world never drink cow's milk (the ideal nutriment for calves!). These people enjoy better health and have better teeth and bones than most Americans. Despite the propaganda of the milk industry, calcium is not exclusively found in milk, but it is plentiful in beans, whole grains, and many vegetables (which do not contain the sugar [lactose] or the damaging fat of whole milk). If you wish to include dairy products in your diet, use low-fat milk, *small* amounts of unsalted butter, and low-fat, unsalted cheese free from chemical additives. Avoid homogenized milk, which makes fat globules smaller and absorbable and is a major factor in the increasing incidence of heart disease.

Meat and Eggs

Cardiologist Kurt Oster, M.D., has found that the enzyme xanthine oxidase, found in homogenized milk damages the heart and clogs the arteries and wants the process changed. Prudence suggests we leave cows' milk in its udderly delicious state for calves.[29] Remember: The healthy peoples of the world eat small amounts of fish, fowl and meat. Protein? Did you ever see a weak gorilla? On a *proper* vegetarian diet, you obtain a proper amount of protein.

---

[28] K. A. Oster, *Myocardiology; Recent Advanced Studies in Cardiac Structure and Metabolism*, Vol. I, University Park Press, Baltimore, 1973.

[29] James F. Balch, M.D., and Phyllis Balch, C.N.C., *Prescription For Nutritional Healing*, Avery Publishing Group, Inc., Garden City Park, N.Y., p. 129.

Avoid fatty meats entirely, and eat less quantities of chicken and fish (but more of beans and grains) for your main dish. The famous Pritikin diet limits meat to ¼ pound daily—only very lean meat or fowl. This means no lamb, pig, duck, shrimp, shellfish, franks, sausages, bacon, or organ meats. Since even fowl and lean meats are often contaminated with pesticides and possibly carcinogenic hormones such as stilbesterol, it is wiser to have seafood occasionally, free range fowl or organically raised meats.

Eggs for some people are banned because of their high cholesterol content. On the other hand, some nutritionists feel that eggs are an ideal food, pointing out that eggs contain lecithin to counteract the cholesterol. If you do eat eggs, limit your intake to a half dozen per week, and if possible, procure them from organically raised free range hens living healthy lives with attentive roosters which lay *fertilized* eggs.

If you still think that you need animal flesh to be strong, remember that increasing numbers of long-distance runners and Olympic athletes are switching to low protein, high complex carbohydrate diets. Perhaps they have heard of the Hunzas of the Himalayas or Tarahumara Indians of Mexico, who have boundless energy. Their wooden kickball races cover 180 miles in forty-eight hours; they run several hundred miles in five days, and they eat meat perhaps only ten times a year along with their 80-10-10 diet of corn, beans, squash, peas, etc. How would you like to join their games after you have consumed fatty hamburgers, white rolls, and chocolate milkshakes?

Bread and Grains

Bread was once the staff of life, until milling, shelf life, and processing made it a wonder of technology—and a

walking stick to the grave. Without fiber, with a few synthetic vitamins replacing the natural goodness that has been
removed, how else can one describe white bread? Health
food stores sell stone-ground whole grain breads, but if you
purchase them make sure that they do not contain sugar
and chemicals. Check the small print on the package ingre-
dients that are not in the master plan for the nourishment of
your body. Better yet, bake your own bread, or ask your
local baker to bake real bread.

Whole grains, organically raised without additives, can
also be purchased at health food stores. They can be slow
cooked overnight with beans and vegetables to preserve
nutrients, and they make wonderful casseroles and soups.

Salt

The average American consumes dangerous amounts of
salt. Experts estimate that one in six persons will develop
fatal high blood pressure, partly due to excess salt intake.[30]
For many thousands of years, the human system was geared
to a low-salt and high-potassium diet of vegetables and
fruits. A high-salt diet throws this balance out of kilter and
causes a buildup of fluid in the tissues, leading to high blood
pressure. This hypertension often leads to kidney damage
and stroke, and it is a factor in heart disease. A low-salt regimen is also beneficial to women in alleviating premenstrual
symptoms such as bloating, headaches, and moodiness.

One can eliminate these poisonous amounts of salt by
avoiding packaged foods, meats, canned soups, processed
cheeses, and cakes (which are loaded with salt as well as
sugar). Substitute herbs and powdered or fresh garlic as

---

[30] Balch, op. cit. p. 204.

seasonings. If you must use salt, small amounts of kelp powder, which contains about forty minerals, is preferable to commercial table salt, which contains dextrose as a stabilizer for added iodine, sodium bicarbonate for whiteness, and an anticaking aluminum to render the salt free-flowing.

Desserts and Beverages

Sorry folks, so am I, but no sugary dessert, pastry, fruit in syrup, or ice cream has a place in the healthy diet. For better digestion and assimilation, it is better to eat fresh whole fruit between meals unless you are hypoglycemic. Raw sunflower seeds, pumpkin seeds, unsalted nuts (in small quantities due to their fat content), and dried, unsulphured fruits, unless you must avoid sugar, make healthy between-meal snacks.

Regular or diet sodas are loaded with sugar and additives, respectively, and should be avoided like the plague. Drink herb teas such as linden, green, rosehips, and alfalfa rather than coffee, which is dangerous because of the effects of caffeine. If you must have coffee, avoid the ones that are chemically decaffeinated; there is now one available that uses a nonchemical process to remove the caffeine, and is available in health food stores.

Be an Organic Windowsill Gardener

Even if you live in a city apartment, it is still possible to enjoy a daily supply of natural, garden-grown food—full of vitamins, minerals, enzymes, and fiber and free of pesticides—for pennies a day. All you need are several quart-size jars. Put a dozen small nail holes in the metal covers, or use cheese cloth held in place over the rims of the jars with rubber bands. Soak about an inch of wheat, oak, alfalfa seeds, or mung beans, in two inches of water for one day. Each day thereafter, add fresh, tepid water and drain through the holes in the tops. Keep your crop moist — neither wet nor dry. When grains and seeds are sprouted, they increase their vitamin and enzyme content as much as 2,000 percent! After sprouting begins, place your jars in the light. Use bottled water if your supply is fluoridated, and remember to buy seeds and natural grains, free of fungicides such as mercury. Other grains and seeds to experiment with are unhulled sesame, sunflower, millet, clover, parsley, wheat, rye, oats, barley, lentils, and lima beans. Many health centers (such as The Hippocrates Center in Boston), use the healing power of wheatgrass in their wholistic programs.

Sprouts may be kept refrigerated, ready to use in soups, salads, casseroles, and vegetable stews. They are best eaten raw — the best living food in the world!

The Syntonic approach to nutrition is not another fad diet, but a way of eating healthy foods that will help you live vigorously as many as perhaps thirty years longer than the current degenerative disease regimen. It has been proven by thousands of years of human experience, and by anthropological studies of healthy societies mentioned before where 100 years is a normal life span. Such a nutrition plan will help you find and maintain your normal weight, lower food costs up to 50 percent, lessen or eliminate dentist and doctor bills, and improve your health and vitality. By avoiding the destructive pseudofoods glorified by clever advertising, you will help yourself avoid the rampant spread of certain killer diseases, drugs, surgery, chemotherapy, and radiation.

Your energy level will increase and your trillions of cells will be cleaner and freer of enervating toxins. Emotionally you will be more balanced, since your glands, organs, and nervous system will function better free of the stress created by sugar and excess meat. The quality of your life—mentally, physically, emotionally, and spiritually—will be enhanced. As Syntonics makes clear, it all goes together!

Summary: Fifteen Ways to Improve Your Health and Happiness through Proper Nutrition

- When tired or not feeling well, rest and abstain from food until your appetite returns.

- When emotionally or mentally upset, do not eat. First use the self-help methods discussed in the last three sections of this book to regain your center and inner balance.

- Follow a prudent diet high in fiber-rich natural foods: whole grains, beans, vegetables, fruits, (unless hypoglycemic) nuts, and seeds. Minimize animal foods and choose seafoods rather than meat.

- As a general rule, eat the whole fruit rather than only the juice. In an orange, for example, the discarded pulp contains more calcium, magnesium, and potassium than the juice.

- Avoid chemical additives and the white plague: white sugar, white bread, white flour, white rice, and salt.

- Use herbs and garlic and onion salt for seasoning, and cold-pressed oils, lemon, herbs, low-fat yogurt, and apple cider vinegar (not wine vinegar) for salad dressings.

- Avoid all desserts. (Long range well-being is better than immediate gratification!)

- For better digestion, even fresh fruit should be eaten between meals rather than immediately following them.

- Avoid tea and coffee (caffeine) and sodas, colas, and low-cal soft drink concoctions (sugar and chemicals). If you must have coffee, use the kind that is decaffeinated with a water process rather than chemicals. Better yet, find herb teas that are nutritious and caffeine free.

- Raise your own organic food. If you are a city dweller, you can still have your own organic garden of sprouted grains and seeds.

- Make sure you are only using pure water, either by purchasing it or using a reverse osmosis machine.

- Avoid hydrogenated fats and oils like the plague (i.e., margarine and other processed crackers, cookies, etc.). The increase of heart disease and cancer has not only been accompanied by increased consumption of animal fat but by a vast increase in the use of oils transformed into trans-fatty acids. Use real natural flax oil, olive oil, and canola oil and avoid the artificial low-cholesterol oils and chemically altered "nonfoods."

- As you move toward a healthy Syntonic diet, get a couple of colonics for a colon cleansing. I also take a spoonful of psyllium powder every morning in a cup of carrot juice. This helps the alimentary canal function properly. Remember, a clogged colon results in self-poisoning, poor assimilation, and a host of unpleasant diseases. You will feel great and thank me for your feeling of lightness and cleanliness.

- Proper food combining can add to proper digestion, assimilation, and general ease and well-being. In nature, animals tend to eat one food at a time. The ideal is to eat and savor foods that can be digested together easily. Experiment with the chart on page 51 and see if you don't feel lighter and better due to more compatible food combinations.

- Remember that alcohol, caffeine, sugar, and white flour not only disturb the blood sugar balance of the body, but they also deplete your body of needed vitamins. This is particularly true of the B vitamins, the lack of which, like hypoglycemia, can create most of the symptoms of neurosis: anxiety, depression, weakness, poor appetite, insomnia, and hostility. Psychotherapy will never work with these biochemical disturbances. This B complex deficiency syndrome is usually misdiagnosed. In Syntonics, we get the body well through proper diet and lifestyle *as well* as treating psychological, emotional, and spiritual inadequacies!

Switching to whole grains takes care of the problem, since they are a prime source of the B vitamins. I also use and recommend brewer's yeast flakes (a health store item) and add it to my oatmeal or sugar-free granola. Don't fall for the hype about "enriched" cereal with synthetic vitamins added. Real vitamins come from nature and natural sources.

The best source I know of for high quality vitamin and mineral supplements in the New York area is The Atkins Center for Complementary Medicine at 152 E. 55 Street. Unless you raise all your foods organically, it is wise to supplement even an ideal diet with Dr. Atkins' Basic Formula

#1, 3 to 6 a day. If you have been hurt or not helped by conventional medicine, the Center affords an evaluation and a personalized program that help your body overcome disease by building health naturally starting with the maxim of Hippocrates; "First do no harm."

On the West Coast, Dr. Julian Whitaker's Wellness Institute in Newport Beach, California, also offers high quality supplements and also has helped thousands reverse the effects of heart disease, arthritis, diabetes, and many other diseases, naturally.

For other areas of the U.S. see "Your Guide to Unconventional Physicians and Therapists after Appendix V.

Syntonic Food Combining for Easiest Digestion

One food at a meal is the most ideal for the easiest and best digestion. Combination of several foods at a meal should follow the chart below. A meal should not consist of more than four foods.

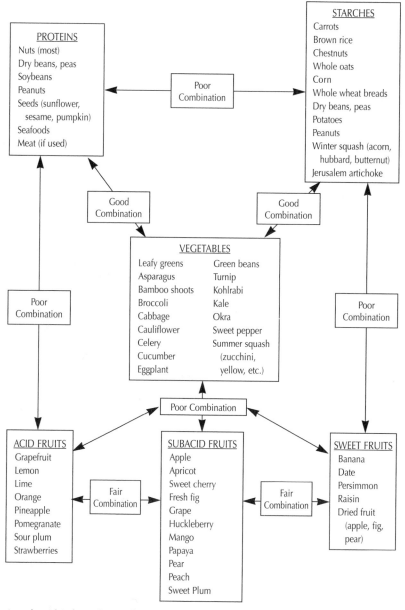

STARCHES
Carrots
Brown rice
Chestnuts
Whole oats
Corn
Whole wheat breads
Dry beans, peas
Potatoes
Peanuts
Winter squash (acorn, hubbard, butternut)
Jerusalem artichoke

PROTEINS
Nuts (most)
Dry beans, peas
Soybeans
Peanuts
Seeds (sunflower, sesame, pumpkin)
Seafoods
Meat (if used)

Poor Combination

Good Combination

Good Combination

VEGETABLES
Leafy greens   Green beans
Asparagus   Turnip
Bamboo shoots   Kohlrabi
Broccoli   Kale
Cabbage   Okra
Cauliflower   Sweet pepper
Celery   Summer squash
Cucumber   (zucchini,
Eggplant   yellow, etc.)

Poor Combination

Poor Combination

Poor Combination

ACID FRUITS
Grapefruit
Lemon
Lime
Orange
Pineapple
Pomegranate
Sour plum
Strawberries

Fair Combination

SUBACID FRUITS
Apple
Apricot
Sweet cherry
Fresh fig
Grape
Huckleberry
Mango
Papaya
Pear
Peach
Sweet Plum

Fair Combination

SWEET FRUITS
Banana
Date
Persimmon
Raisin
Dried fruit
  (apple, fig, pear)

Avocados, rich in fat, are best combined with green vegetables.
Tomatoes may be best eaten with nonstarchy vegetables and proteins.

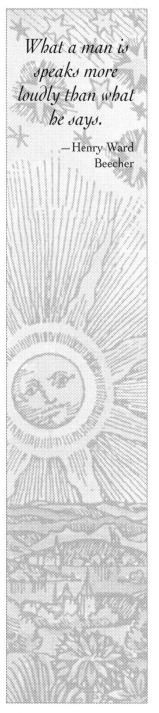

THREE

Freeing Your Body from Chronic Tension

The accumulated experience of human beings with self-awareness and awareness of others has produced many insights concerning the human body. Such insights focus on various parts of the body and the ways in which muscular tensions are connected with destructive emotional and mental attitudes. Since the emotions, the mind, and the body are parts of a whole, body tensions, feelings, and thoughts are all interrelated. For this reason, wholistic

53

Syntonic therapy is more effective since it works with all dimensions of the person.

It is my aim in this chapter to enumerate chronic areas of tension and to indicate ways in which you can help release these tensions. Release of tension is an important part of total therapy and of self-reeducation.

Unfortunately, many psychotherapies omit the roles of physical health, nutrition, and tension from the therapeutic process. Therapists who have been trained psychologically have a fear and resistance to considering tensions of the body in their therapeutic work. Even the word *psychotherapy* indicates a partial approach and a split between mind and body. To my knowledge, no one has found a physiological line of demarcation between the two. The Syntonic therapy [1] which I have developed combines Freud's psychoanalytic insights; Wilhelm Reich's work with character analysis; breathing and muscular tension; guided fantasy techniques; catharsis through sounds and movements; neural linguistic programing; change of diet and living habits; and the spiritual wisdom contained in yoga and world religions.

Enjoying Deeper, Fuller Breathing

The idea that breath is life is as old as the yoga and Hindu traditions. In the Bible, in Genesis it is written that "the Lord God molded man out of the dust of the ground and breathed into his nostrils the breath of life." Healthy breathing and movement are the essence of life. It is foolish to overlook these factors in the therapeutic process. I have

---

[1] *Syntonic,* the name of this total therapy, means integrating *(syn)* the energy vibrations *(tonic)* of the organism into a positive, loving flow.

worked with many patients whose previous and often lengthy therapy or psychoanalysis left them intellectually aware—yet still discouraged, alienated, or desperate because their breathing, movements, sensations, and emotions had not been liberated.

The ancient Greeks stressed the importance of a sound mind in a sound body. A sound body in my view is one that is vital and robust. Its breathing is unimpaired and it produces adequate energy. It glows and has warmth. Further, a sound body has ease rather than dis-ease and free, graceful, flowing movements that are the outward sign of inner pleasure. To possess grace is to be in touch with the Life Force (that is, God's grace). Bodies that are twisted and bound up or segmented by deep tensions are dammed up reservoirs of intense fear, chronic sadness, and rage. The fruits of the Spirit, when you feel your true nature as wholeness (holiness), are love, hope, and faith.

A third characteristic of a sound body is that it is balanced and well grounded. These terms show the wisdom of language, for we speak of people who have their feet on the ground in the sense that they are "with it" (in contact with reality) rather than "out of it," "off the wall," "up in the clouds," or "spaced out." *A sound body is centered two inches below the navel* and has vitality which flows in a graceful and pleasurable way. When you are centered with your weight underneath, you have a secure feeling of being grounded and down to earth. Such physical and emotional well-being is essential for sound and realistic thinking and for a wholeness of personality. Its disturbance is accompanied by varying degrees of mental instability, irrational anxiety, fears, doubts, self-blame, grandiosity and worthlessness, psychopathic rationalization and behavior, and the projection of unacceptable feelings onto others. Beginning on page 67 of this book, I describe a centering technique which helps to unify the mind and body.

The Body Speaks—What Is Yours Saying?

Irrational thinking creates negative emotions and physical tensions, and vice versa. Thus, total therapy *must* change both mental and physical attitudes! In helping yourself toward inner peace, all parts of your life are involved. Fears and doubts begin early.

Freud's psychoanalytic insight into the human development process and the importance of the oral (first) stage of development is validated by folk wisdom. As Drs. Spitz and Leboyer[2] have shown, early infantile psychological disturbance creates a predisposition for later mental illness. Mental disturbance is described (nonverbally) by the gesture of the forefinger pointed at the temple and rotated in a small circle; this gesture indicates that the mind is disturbed by excessive energy and "crazy" thinking. Verbal descriptions of mental illness refer to "bats in the belfry" and to individuals "in a world of their own" or who are "not with it"—that is, not with their own body and its emotions (this is sometimes called depersonalization).

The insecure child often becomes the severely dependent and weak adult who "hangs on like a leech," is "on the bottle" (it is estimated that there are as many as twelve million alcoholics in America), "doesn't have two legs to stand on," or has "cold feet" (fear) in relation to other people and to life. The exercises which will be described in this book—

---

[2] Dr. René Spitz. *The First Year of Life,* Internat. Universities Press, N.Y., 1965 pp. 199-208. Dr. Frederick LeBoyer, *Birth Without Violence,* Alfred A. Knopf, N.Y., 1980.

such as positive anger and stamping—are designed to help increase assertiveness and strengthen emotional security.

In religious psychology, "stiff-necked pride" is the cardinal sin which separates one from contact with God, the Life Force, and the feeling of love for one's fellows. Real pride or self-respect comes from feeling one's warmth and aliveness. Being "above it all" and having a "stubborn jaw" or a "thick head" also describe the physical aspect of psychological disturbances such as arrogance and unreasonableness. The neck, jaw, and breathing exercises we will discuss will help you overcome these self-defeating attitudes.

What Do *Your* Eyes Express?

The eyes have been rightly called the windows of the soul, for they are the most important organ of contact with the material world and communicate the inner state of one's being. Eyes express all emotions and attitudes and can appear dead, blank, lively, far away, scared, terrified, angry, cold, hateful, warm, suspicious, innocent, diabolical, searching, seductive, shifty, honest, guilty, lost, sad, hopeless, amazed, defiant, etc. Chronically dilated pupils reveal severe emotional disturbance, and careful observation reveals that eyes wax and wane in their intensity of color, depending on the level of aliveness, breathing, and feeling in the person. (Similarly, colors fade on a dolphin or tuna after it is boated.) Frequently after a dynamic Syntonic total therapy session, clients will remark that everything looks brighter, and indeed their eyes will appear more alive and colorful!

The upper back and shoulders are also crucial areas in which we maintain emotional and psychological negativity. The expression that someone is "hung up" describes extreme tension in this area, which can greatly damage the capacity to reach assertively and lovingly toward the world. Very sick people often identify with the image of Jesus on the Cross, whereas many healthy people draw inspiration from Jesus the whole man of love, faith, and courage. To have one's "back up" is a phrase that describes negative thinking, general mistrust, and sometimes the feeling of being followed. One is, in fact, being followed by that fear and anger caught in one's tense neck and back!

Energies normally mobilized through fear, anger, and rage (often in the early layers of the personality) become frozen within such deep tensions. The person with a "chip on his shoulder" who chronically holds his "back up" is ready for a fight and often manages to provoke one. Such attitudes have been part of the emotional epidemic which has plagued humankind since the fall from grace described in the Bible. They comprise the demonic element which destroys the peace of countless families, transmits emotional illness through generations, and feeds racial and religious prejudice to the extremes of genocide and international warfare.

The upward and outward flow of feeling toward the world can also be blocked by tensions in the front of the body. We often speak of the need to "get something off our chest," or the feeling of being "down in the mouth" when emotions of fear, sadness, and/or anger are arrested by deep inner tension and swallowed down. Compulsive eaters attack food and swallow down such feelings. The terms *warm hearted* or *cold hearted* denote the flow or repression of loving feelings in the chest area. We have discovered in our wholistic therapy that the use of sounds is an important part of emotional release, to express fear, sadness, rage, or pleasure that go beyond words.

Deep tensions in the upper body, which start with frustration and deprivation in the nursing phase of child development, have a disastrous effect on the pleasure, growth, and well-being of the whole organism. In adulthood these tensions bind fear, despair, and rage in the individual and transform the natural feeling of self-esteem and enthusiasm for life into guilt, meaninglessness, and ennui. The ability to draw a free breath, which neurotic and psychotic individuals cannot do, becomes a stolen birthright.

Premature toilet training (before the infant is ready to regulate itself) and prudish, antisexual attitudes give rise to further tension in the body. In adulthood this leads to added underlying anxiety (so common as to be called "basic") and a variety of sexual, emotional, and mental disturbances.[3] Breathing and tension-release exercises in our Syntonic therapy help the outward flow of energy and physical and spiritual expansion.

Deep pelvic tensions block the feelings of warm and loving sexuality, resulting in overall tension and inhibited breathing, "mechanical sex," "cold" men and "frigid" women, and varying degrees of impotence. In addition, history and contemporary life are full of examples of people who lack the "guts" or courage to stand for what is decent, which stems from warm caring and loving emotions. The phrase "bowels of compassion" describes people who can feel for others in contrast to those who are "tight assed," uncaring, and unforgiving. The goose stepping Nazis were perfect examples of cold, mechanical, sadistic, psychopathic and cowardly murderers; fear and love are opposite sides of the autonomic nervous system. (See Personality Chart.)

---

[3] See the Personality Chart.

Frozen Heart, Frozen Pelvis

The vernacular for human genitals expresses a derogatory attitude toward the body. Four-letter words that refer to the genitals demean and insult men and women. The word *prick*, defined in my office dictionary as "a pointed instrument or weapon," has a hostile connotation and is used as an insult to a man. The fear (coldness) and hostility (tension) that underlie ungratifying intercourse, whether homosexual or heterosexual, are described in the "F" word. This word has a very different meaning than the sexuality described by the term *making love*. Women and men suffering from varying degrees of nymphomania and satyromania (who are seeking to release feelings that are blocked by their bodily tensions) are chronically promiscuous until they find the capacity to relax and find fulfillment through therapeutic aid or self-help.

Promiscuity is not uncommon in immature marriage relationships, although the promiscuity is often on a fantasy level, imagining someone other than one's partner during unsatisfactory intercourse. D. H. Lawrence was aware of the tragic result of the destructive education of so-called civilized man. In an essay titled "Obscenity and Pornography," he wrote that "the sickness of our civilization is the great lie of purity and the dirty little secret, and in this lie the money lie hides." Spoil the wholeness and the freedom and the flow of the Life Force that is love, turn us against our bodies and souls with irrational fear and neurotic guilt, and what is left but the attempt to gain pseudosecurity and self-respect by accumulating material possessions?

No one put it better than Wilhelm Reich who said in a seminar, "The trouble with the world is that there is too much f---ing, (I would say literally and figuratively mis-using others in *all* areas of human intercourse) and too little loving."

The lower half of the body, from the pelvis down, often suffers more problems of feeling and contact than does the upper half. Many women have more feeling in kissing than in intercourse, and some will be very particular about whom they kiss but indiscriminate about having sex. Many men are far more aware of their tongue than of their penis. Orality is overplayed to the extent that true sexuality is underdeveloped. In the full and loving sexual union, the sense of an individual separate self and consciousness is overcome so that, with one's lover, one is carried beyond time and space to return to a sense of rebirth. This is the *mysterium tremendum* which is as different from the common variety of puritanical-pornographic-mechanical sex as wheat from chaff. Those who have been free enough and loving enough to experience this know the deep meaning of the expression, "It's bigger than both of us."

Everyone, on some level, both longs for and is afraid of love. The core of our being, as observed in every normal infant, is to reach out and respond to life appreciatively and lovingly—unless outer reality is threatening or the inner flow is curtailed. Unfortunately for most of humanity, it is no more possible to make love truly with a tense body than it is to caress someone with a clenched fist. Without opening one's heart and risking the pain that may result, one cannot love. Only the "lionhearted" (Gilbert and Sullivan wrote that "faint heart never won fair lady") can know one of the greatest experiences of life.

A nervous and immature married woman met with a wise and famous preacher named Harry Emerson Fosdick of the Riverside Church in New York City. She confessed that she could not believe in and experience God. Knowing that this meant that she was disconnected from her deeper emotions and being, he replied; "I suggest you get therapeutic help;

there's something wrong with your sex life."

The belly and solar plexus (colloquially the "pit of the stomach") are the centers of feeling and emotion. Intense fear can paralyze us like a blow to the solar plexus. A person who is chronically afraid is described lacking "intestinal fortitude." During the state of fear, there is a strong contraction of the body and viscera. If fear overcomes one completely, one freezes in a state of terror. A stronger person can breathe through fear and mobilize energy to fight, if necessary. The hero possesses guts, courage to overcome fear, and the ability to act. The pseudohero denies and represses fear and often does not remember what happened. Chronic deprivation of love through childhood creates generalized fear or anxiety, often called "butterflies in the stomach," describing energy that is neither bound up nor able to flow out through expression. This is the state of anxious anticipation, of indecision. (See the Personality Chart.)

Dependent individuals (those who are orally fixated and immature and who are masochistic and addictive personalities) often cannot "stomach" experiences, but swallow them meekly or "grin and bear" them. The former type are too weak to do anything but occasionally yell desperately and cling like fearful children. The latter smirk and sneer as a defense (contempt on the Personality Chart) but are bound up in their guts and lack the "backbone" to be assertive. More aggressive or phallic types may show aggression, thus camouflaging the fear and tension which prevent them from the ability to compromise, to be reasonable, to apologize, or to love.

The weak, spiteful, and the tough tend to be "uptight." The weak have little to give, for their breath and energy are fragile. The masochistic and spiteful *won't* give, for they are bound up in self-destructive tension and negativity. Tough and aggressive men and women are afraid to soften and yield their armor, and can only take from others.

"To fall in love" means that one's heart is touched; one feels deeply moved and excited. This deep feeling of love, (symbolized by Cupid), which infants have with their mother, is reactivated in our maturity when we feel that we have found our beloved! Those who never had that warmth and closeness as infants ("the milk of human kindness") are too tense and afraid to fall in love, denying the very existence of love. For them God is dead, and love is dead.

With a disunified body, low level of energy, and constricted breathing, one cannot experience the Life Force, just as one cannot light a lamp that is not plugged into the energy source. For this reason, religious or rational arguments about the meaning of existence are merely verbal acrobatics. One may as well try to convince a depressed person that life can be beautiful. Having "sold their souls to the devil," many people have withdrawn into hospitals, their own fantasies, or the psychopathic pursuit of material and sexual power. Lacking an inner spirit of aliveness, they sneer at faith, mock hope, and despairingly or spitefully deny that life has any meaning or value.

Many of us are neurotic individuals who have had some taste of warmth and "the milk of human kindness," but not enough. Our hearts are not frozen, but timid. Ambivalence or "chicken-heartedness" characterizes such people, who *wish* to feel strongly but are unable to, because their tensions block the flow of pleasure—causing them to experience, in Wilhelm Reich's term, "pleasure anxiety."[4] If they begin to

---

[4] Wilhelm Reich, M.D., *Character Analysis*, Orgone Inst. Press., N.Y., 1949, Chap. XIV.

feel the inner warmth and flow of expansive feelings, they become afraid and quickly rationalize that "I'll be caught," "I'll become too dependent and lose myself," or "I'm unworthy, so how could anyone love me in return, and if they do, there must be something wrong with them." If such neurotic people are aware of having angry or aggressive feelings, they hold back for fear of losing control. This is a common and valid fear among tense, neurotic individuals, who periodically explode and then guiltily return to a subsequent period of suppression. Syntonic therapy offers exercises in emotional release that are designed to change this blocked rage into a positive therapeutic force.

Rather than face fear, most neurotics deny it or seek to escape it through alcohol, drugs, or promiscuity. When feeling pain or sadness, they "grin and bear it" or choke down their tears and flee from their emotions.

Deep sexual feelings are as feared as they are longed for. To go into the "deep blue sea" of emotions demands the faith and courage to surrender to the involuntary movements and the deep breathing of true passion, a power likened to the force of tidal waves in dreams. The "fainthearted" retreat into watchfulness for safety against losing control, as they believe "better be safe than sorry." Contrast this with the affirmative attitude: "Nothing ventured, nothing gained."

There is a direct connection between chronic bodily tensions and self-defeating thinking, feeling, and behavior. The daily exercise program outlined in the next chapter will help you free yourself from your tensions.

Gradually you will find yourself becoming more relaxed, more aware of your center, and more in touch with the Life Energy. Living will become joyful and meaningful, and each day will become not a burden, but a challenging adventure!

Points to Remember About the Physical Tensions and the Emotional and Mental Disturbances That Sabotage Human Health and Happiness

- A wholistic approach to therapy is important.
- Breathing and movement are basic living functions.
- The healthy state of being is centered and grounded.
- Nonviolent, natural childbirth and intimate bonding and nursing satisfaction are crucial for infant and mother.
- There is a connection between folk expressions, different parts of the body, and pathological attitudes and behavior.
- There is a relationship between infantile experience and adult sexual and emotional disturbances.
- Prevention is necessary to deal with the emotional plague of psychosomatic illness, delinquency, corruption, crime, addiction, and neuroses.
- There is an interrelationship among physical tension, irrational thinking, negative emotions, and stagnant spirituality.
- Specific daily exercises are important to relax physically and thereby enhance one's total well-being. (These are described in the following chapter.)

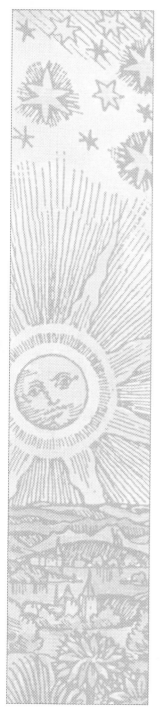

F O U R

A Healthier, More Vital You

Since toxemia and tension are the two great enemies of our physical well-being, a healthy diet along with the exercises discussed in the chapter will yield great rewards in increased health, vitality, and energy flow.

Physical Exercises to Start the Day

Let us begin now to lessen physical tension and to move in the direction of healthful relaxation. Assume a position on your knees on your bed. Sit on your heels with the soles of your feet upward. If this begins to hurt, occasionally rise onto your knees and continue the exercises. Gradually you will be able to sit on your heels for longer periods of time as the muscles of your feet, ankles, and legs become freer of tension. Maintain a straight back: Imagine a plumb line rising from your lower back up through your neck and head.

Breath

Focus on a point two inches below your navel and breathe gently into that area. Feel your abdomen expand as you breathe in deeply, and release as you exhale. This is the natural way to breathe, and in itself can relieve tension and anxiety. Be aware of breathing this way as much as possible throughout each day, but without strain. This is the way we breathe when we are relaxed and can draw a free breath, or when we heave a sigh of relief. Later in this chapter, we will discuss breathing further.

Scalp

Taking handfuls of hair, gently pull your scalp in different directions. Now move your scalp by raising and lowering the muscles of your forehead. Alternately open your eyes wide, then frown. Gradually you will begin to feel your ears move.

Eyes

Close your eyes tightly and gently press them with the heels of your hand. Move your eyes as far to the left and as far to the right as possible in a horizontal line. Then move your eyes toward the direction of the ceiling and toward the floor. Repeat if you wish, but remember to breathe into your center, below your navel, keeping your awareness there as much as possible.

Head and Neck

Open your mouth and jaw as wide as you can as you inhale. Exhale and relax. Try to touch the tip of your tongue to your nose, then down to your chin, to stretch the muscles of the throat. Exhale and relax. Drop your chin to your chest (your body upright and relaxed). Rotate your chin in a wide, easy circle to the left as you inhale, without moving your shoulders at all. Rotate your head back so that your face is toward the ceiling; just drop the weight of the head easily back. As you exhale, continue moving your head in a circle toward the right. Repeat, gently, rotating your head in the opposite direction. Inhaling through your nose, begin again with the chin on the chest, and so on.

Shoulders

Relax your shoulders by raising them as far as possible toward your ears as you inhale into the center below your navel. Let your shoulders fall back to rest as you exhale, letting the weight of the world fall from your shoulders. Rotate your shoulders back, up, and forward; again, rest as you exhale. Repeat the opposite way: forward, up, back, and again at rest with the exhalation. Shake your shoulders without moving the rest of your trunk. You may find it helpful to practice this in front of a mirror.

Diaphragm

To deepen your breathing and loosen your diaphragm, breathe in with several strong sniffing movements through your nose; and again relax as you exhale. Do this several times. Then let your breath out completely and tighten and loosen your stomach muscles as many times as you can without strain, before inhaling.

Back

On your hands and knees, with arms and thighs vertical, drop your chin to your chest and curl your pelvis in toward your head. Inhale through your nose while moving your head up and back as far as possible as you bring your buttocks up toward the back of your head. In this position, feel the arch stretching your back muscles. As you exhale, bring your head and pelvis back to the curled position. Again, feel the opposite stretching of your back muscles.

Next, lie on your back on a bed. Raise your legs toward the ceiling, supporting your back with your hands so that your weight is on your hands and shoulders and your trunk and legs are in a straight line (see the drawing). Gradually you will be able to achieve this position comfortably. Watch your lower belly move as you breathe in and out. Slowly bring your legs back over your head as far as you can. Your toes eventually will be able to touch the bed with your legs straight. Then raise your legs in the air, and make bicycle movements as long as you wish without strain.

Legs

While on your back, legs and calves relaxed on the bed, tighten your legs by flexing your toes as far toward your head as possible as you inhale; relax your legs completely as you exhale. Now center your awareness below your navel. Breathe easily. Look within to see if there is any area of

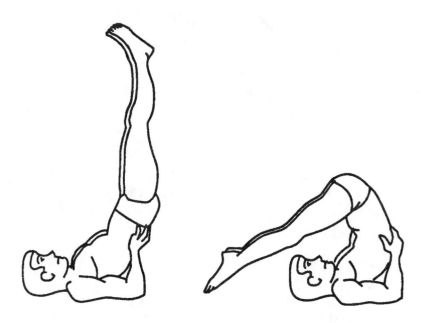

The Candle

The Plow

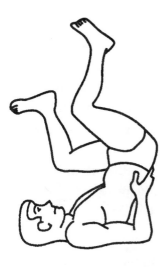

The Bicycle

tension in any part of your body. If so, tighten that part as you inhale, and relax as you exhale.

Take a standing position, with your bare feet about a foot apart and parallel. Again picture a plumb line through your whole body so that it is upright and relaxed. Continue to place your awareness in your center of gravity below the navel. Inhale through your nose, breathing into your whole body. Relax as you exhale, and feel your feet gently rooted into the floor with the top of your head gently upright toward the sky. Feel the contact between the top of your head and the outer cosmos.

To stretch and expand your body further, imagine that you are pushing the ceiling up with your palms; hold for several breaths, and then let your arms and shoulders drop back to the relaxed position. Repeat if you wish. Imagine that you are pushing walls away from each side of your body with your palms; hold for several breaths, and then relax.

Pelvis

With your hands on your hips and your legs slightly bent (they should never be held stiff with knees locked), rotate your pelvis — not your back and thighs, just your pelvis — in as wide a circle as possible. Start in a forward position, inhaling as you move all the way to the back position in a circle, and exhale as you continue around to the forward position again. Alternate several times in the other direction. To discover and free this movement, it helps to practice before a mirror.

Energy

In the same upright position, with knees bent slightly, start a rapid up-and-down movement with your legs, let this rhythmic movement take over, feet firmly planted, and feel your whole body move as if with a built-in vibrator from your ankles all the way to your head. Let this be an automatic movement so that the spring in your legs and knees can shake you free of any other tension of which you might be aware. Let the movement and feeling of energy excitation flow through your whole being.

Now your body will be more relaxed, your breathing more free, and your vitality stronger than when you began these exercises. Each time you do this series, you will increase your physical well-being. As in everything else, the more you give to these exercises, the more you will receive from them.

Embrace Relaxation

It is a basic principle of life that thought directs energy and energy follows thought. After exercising, lie down for a minute or two and focus your attention on deep, easy breathing into your center, just below your navel, and be aware of the easy rhythm of breathing. Mentally examine your body to locate any area of tension. Tighten this area as you inhale. After holding your breath for a count of three, release as you blow the air out. As with your dietary change, proceed gradually and easily.[1]

Bathing

Since your skin is an organ of elimination of toxins, it is desirable to take a shower or bath each morning followed by a brisk rubdown all over your body with a thick towel.

---

[1] A cassette tape is available as a supplement to this program and is designed to help you improve all four dimensions of your well-being (see page ???).

Alimentary Massage

After bathing, bend over slightly, exhale completely, and press firmly with your fingertips from just above the pubic bone. Then make a circle up the right side, around under your ribs, and down the left side. This stimulates the energy flow through your colon and is helpful in promoting elimination. Remember, if you fail to get rid of the toxins in your body, they will get rid of you.

Breathe Into Every Cell

Breathing fresh air into all parts of your lungs is as important as such daily exercise as walking, cycling, swimming, and playing tennis or other sports that do not overtax your body. Breath is life. We actually bring the Life Force (called *prana* in India, *ki* in Japan, and *chi* in China) into our bodies. We can live many weeks without food and a few days without water, but very few seconds without air.

Most people have been conditioned to breathe shallowly up in the chest, which is part of a tense, anxious, and watchful attitude. To reeducate ourselves toward a relaxed state of physical well-being, we must learn to breathe as nature intended. Watch any animal or infant breathe and you will see that their breath begins in the center below the navel and rises through the ribs and chest.

This is so unusual for most of us that we only breathe this way when we heave a sigh of relief, after some particularly tense situation. Gradually train yourself to breathe this way until you reestablish this natural way of breathing and can enjoy a current of energy flowing through you with every exhalation. All natural functions of the body, when done in harmony with the laws of the universe, are pleasurable.

Unless there is a realistic outer cause for fear or pain, a healthy body should be a constant souce of vitality, pleasure, and joy.

Remember that health means doing things with ease and avoiding dis-ease. Inhale as gently and deeply as if you were smelling a beautiful rose, and exhale with a relaxed feeling of letting your breath go to the ends of the universe.

Enhancing Your Sleep

Adequate sleep is just as important for well-being as proper exercise and nutrition, adequate sunlight, fresh air, exercise, and pure water. Sleep, the marvelous balm of which poets speak, is necessary so the "inner physician" can repair your body and maintain the work of digestion, assimilation, and elimination. Every one of our trillions of cells must perform the process of ingestion and drainage. Billions of cells die and must be replaced. Without adequate sleep, these processes are impeded, undermining the body's crucial functions. Experiments have shown that continued sleep deprivation for several days results in bizarre and psychotic symptoms. In countries and institutions where human life is denigrated, depriving a person of sleep is used as a form of torture.

The best sleep reflects the laws of nature, in harmony with the setting and rising of the sun (as the adage says, "Early to bed and early to rise, makes a man healthy, wealthy, and wise."). Obviously, you cannot be "healthy, wealthy, and wise" if you are habitually a nightowl. If you gradually change to a healthier sleep pattern, at least on nights when it is not essential to stay up late, you will add another plus on the side of health and happiness.

Your quality of sleep is enhanced by fresh air and warm

but light covering. In sleep as in everything, the law of moderation is important. Avoid being too warm or too cold, be balanced as in all aspects of your life. Balance and love are essentially interfused with one another. Love is involved with creativity, harmony, growth, and joy. Balance is also a dynamic equilibrium of forces, avoiding extremes and creating a harmony between different energies. On the cosmic level, in growth there is a balance between expansion *(yin)* and contraction or order *(yang)*. On the personal level, is not a loving person a balanced person, both receptive and assertive (both for himself or herself and for others in appropriate ways)?

If insomnia is one of your problems, remember that insomnia (as with all symptoms) is an indication of violations of the orderly processes of life. As in all areas of life, the law of *karma* (we reap what we sow) is immutable. So do not take chemical poisons or alcohol to deaden your system in order to "get a good night's sleep." Rather, consider Socrates' teaching which I learned in college, "The unexamined life is not worth living." Focus attention on slow, deep breathing. Examine the areas of your life in which you are violating the principles of health and happiness and remember that your symptoms will be cured, not just suppressed, if you discover and remove the cause or causes.

It will also help along the way if you do some of the emotional, mental, and spiritual exercises as described in later chapters to quiet the mind.

Remember that exercise during the day and healthy eating patterns before retiring (heavy meat eating is stressful and indulging in sugar and sweets creates tension and anxiety) are conducive to peaceful rest. Nutrients such as calcium (300 mg.), niacinamide (200 mg.) and magnesium (75 mg.) can be helpful. The best bodily exercise I have found to overcome insomnia is to tighten separate areas of your body as you inhale, holding your breath and tension for a count of three, and then relaxing as you exhale.

When Ingrid came to me for a therapeutic "tune-up" for her life, one of her symptoms was insomnia. As with so many of us in this society, Ingrid was full of physical, emotional, and mental toxins, and among a myriad of other symptoms, she was unable to sleep. She gave up sleeping pills because she sensed they were damaging her body, but she drank vodka instead to deaden her tension and anxiety. In the morning she needed several cups of strong coffee to "get going."

Several therapy sessions and a three-day fast followed by healthy nutrition taught Ingrid how to release her pain and nervousness and strengthen her healthy self. As she learned to focus on her center, below the navel, she was able to fall asleep easily by quieting her mind, have a refreshing rest, and wake up feeling better than she dreamed possible. As she continued a new and healthy way of life, she amazed herself and her friends with her rejuvenation.

A beautiful and peaceful night's sleep will be disturbed by caffeine, nicotine and alcohol which have much the same disturbing effect as sugar. Try a "Sleepy Time" herbal tea from the health food store.

Food Combining

Different foods require different digestive processes. The ideal for a happy stomach and easy digestion is to eat and savor foods that can be digested together in good combinations. Although this may be difficult to arrange at all times, wherever possible you will find it worth the effort. Find the way that is most comfortable for you.

Allergies—Helping Yourself through Elimination Dieting

As a wholistic therapist in private practice and as former director of the New Horizon Wholistic Health Center, I have occasionally seen patients suffering from an endless array of physical, emotional, mental, and behavioral symptoms, the causes of which remained a mystery. These hapless individuals usually had a long history of conventional medical evaluations, hospitalization, and sometimes extended psychiatric treatment based on the theory that their ailments were psychosomatic. They had tried a variety of medications that not only failed to help, but often exacerbated symptoms—or even caused damaging side-effects (iatrogenic disease).

The reasons for these symptoms proved to be severe allergic reactions to certain intolerable foods, as well as certain medications which had a toxic effect on the body. In 400 B.C., Hippocrates warned against the medications of his time and counseled, "Let your food be your medicine." And we still paraphrase the aphrorism of Lucretius: "What is food to one man may be fierce poison to others." It is imperative, that we find out how many of our psychiatric patients are victims of chemicalized and fractured foods.

More recently, my colleague the late Dr. Albert Rowe designed "elimination diets" for patients who suffered from symptoms for which a cause could not be discovered. Such symptoms included fatigue, headache, depression, irritated colon, nasal catarrh, irrational or violent behavior, extreme mood swings, fainting spells, sexual problems, skin disorders, and many others. He would advise his patients to leave certain foods out of their diet—such as citrus fruits, canned foods, cereal foods (breads, cakes, and pastry)—and observe whether their symptoms disappeared.

In one case, a woman developed severe physical and behavioral symptoms after the birth of her third child. She became nauseated, moody, irritable, violent toward her children, and would slash her forearms with sharp objects. She had psychiatric therapy followed by electric shock therapy, and numerous psychotropic drugs.

On the theory that she had become allergic to certain foods, Dr. Rowe put her on a fast for several days. Drinking only pure water and eliminating all foods, she showed a marked improvement physically and emotionally as well as in her mental outlook. Then she was gradually given one food at a time, and her reactions to these foods were carefully monitored. Safe foods caused no negative side effects, but foods that were toxic to her created symptoms — sometimes within a minute or two after they were ingested. Once, after she ate white bread, she hallucinated that a herd of deer were in a parking lot.

Another patient who came to me for Syntonic therapy because of depression, anxiety attacks, aversion to sexual intercourse with his wife, and periods of exhaustion in the middle of the day proved to be another case of food allergy that exacerbated his underlying emotional problems. He had been in extensive analytic and psychiatric treatment that dealt only with his emotional problems without also treating his severe nutritional problems. After a three-day fast, he was introduced to one food at a time at two-hour intervals. He had no problems with fresh fish, but reacted adversely to canned seafoods. He did well with salads, steamed vegetables, and fruits, but could not handle a simultaneous intake of vegetables and fruits. He ate yogurt with impunity but began to feel uncomfortable with milk and cheese. In the same manner, he thrived on eggs and whole grain bread (without preservatives), but white bread, sugar, pastry, ice cream, and coffee produced depression and exhaustion. Once his low blood sugar reaction and aversion to canned seafood, milk, cheese, white bread, sugar, ice cream, caffeine, and chemical additives was righted, his improvement was marked: He regained the energy and will to work out his sexual, emotional, mental, and interpersonal problems through Syntonic therapy.

A nine-year-old boy also needed (in addition to therapy) attention to his food allergies. Hypertense, overactive, and violent in school, Tim was unable to concentrate and disturbed by insomnia, stammering, hand trembling, and nail biting. Because it is difficult to recommend that a youngster undertake fasting, I suggested that all processed foods, sugar, white flour, candy, canned soups, packaged cereals, ice cream, etc. be omitted from his and the family's diet. I saw him three times by himself and twice with his family in therapy to help resolve school and home problems. By eliminating the aforementioned foods, Tim's "incurable" symptoms disappeared from his own and his parents' lives too: Mother suffered from dermatitis and stomach problems and Father had colon problems and chronic sinusitis. In addition, we held family group sessions in which everyone expressed their feelings—positive and negative—to each other in an attempt to resolve family problems concerning daily habits such as bedtime, homework time, etc. A month later when I saw the family for a check-up, I was overjoyed. Energy was flowing in healthy and loving ways, whereas it was once wasted in worry and guilt and twisted in destructive and hostile interactions.

The wholistic way of health and happiness places the responsibility on each of us for our own lives. Try a short fast and eliminate foods that interfere with your well-being. Raise your own food—at least sprouted seeds and grains. Select natural and whole foods free of salt, sugar, fats, and additives. This is our challenge and opportunity. See how your energy level improves as well as your attitude toward everything in your life. Through fasting and the elimination process, you can be your own doctor—a stranger to drugs and surgery— while working with the greatest doctor of all: the "inner physician," the healing power of your own God-given body.

Increasing Sexual Vigor

Genuine sexuality is an expression of inner vitality, of love for another human being, and of surrender to the Life Force itself. Sex is often misused for mere release of tension or as an expression of anger, hostility, or contempt. Often women and men use sex to conquer or control one another and act out their passivity or hostility in a neurotic sexual drama. Genuine sexuality combines passion with tender- ness and always has as its components respect for oneself and one's deep emotions, respect for one's partner and a car- ing for his or her well-being, and a reverence for life: a sense of the beauty, the mystery, and the joy of creation.

Sex and the Body

A body that is tired, tense, and toxic will lack the energy for sexual pleasure and joy. All four dimensions of one's being are involved in vital living, and sexuality is but one branch of the whole tree. Along with the general program of self-fulfillment outlined in these pages, there are specific practices which can help increase sexual vitality.

Chronic muscle tensions in the pelvic area can block sex- ual sensations and energy flow. Breathe in sharply, filling the abdomen *first* and then the ribs and chest. Hold for a count of two—at the same time, tighten the muscles of your pelvis and buttocks and release these muscles as you exhale. By consciously tightening and releasing these muscles, you can gradually learn to relax them. Be aware of your center to eliminate mental distractions, neurotic thinking, doubts, and inhibitions. Picture energy flowing from your center when you are with your partner.

The abdomen is the seat of emotions in the human being. Breathing easily and deeply in the navel area during love making helps release tension and open up deeper feelings.

There is some evidence that sexual inadequacy (impotency in the male, frigidity in the female, and sterility in both) is also related to nutrition. Along with the need for whole, naturally raised, and toxin-free foods, certain vitamins and minerals have a beneficial effect on the sexual glands. Zinc is a mineral that is directly connected with the functioning of the prostrate gland in men. It can be found in a natural form in unroasted and unsalted pumpkin seeds.

In addition, vitamins B, E, and A are all involved in enhancing the functioning of the sexual glands. Seeds, nuts, and whole grains are the best natural sources of B and E. Vitamin E has been called the miracle vitamin, the heart-saver vitamin, and the virility vitamin. It oxygenates the tissues of the body and can prevent degeneration of the germinal cells of the testicles, diminished hormone production, female and male sterility, and destruction of the sex hormones by oxidation. Diminished sex hormone production is responsible for premature aging as well as diminished sexual vitality.

Fresh green vegetables and codliver oil are excellent sources of vitamin A. These vegetables also provide fiber, which is necessary for the proper elimination functions of the body. It is also advisable to use kelp, a ground and dried seaweed, which is rich in iodine and trace elements.

Sexual health and vitality are also enhanced by avoiding excessive intake of fatty animal foods, which cause stress in the body and create toxins in the alimentary canal. Avoid all refined, processed, and unnatural foods (such as those discussed in Chapter 2), which deplete the body of the vitamins, minerals, and enzymes that produce sexual vitality. In addition, alcohol is an antiaphrodisiac. Though it has a disinhibiting effect on our minds, it has a damaging effect on the nervous system and diminishes our potential for sexual potency and pleasure.

Herbs That Can Help Boost Your Libido

Herbs have played an important part in both curing illnesses and building health throughout human history. To enhance sexuality, Siberian ginseng, yohimbe, damiana, foti, gota kola, sarsaparilla, and saw palmetto berries have all been found to be helpful, and a combination of these herbs is often called the "love formula" for its aphrodisiac qualities. (You can obtain this combination from the Health Center for Better Living, 6189 Taylor Road, Naples, FL 33942.)

Herbs work gently and safely without the side-effects and iatrogenic effects of so many medications. Another helpful herb combination is a thirty-day program to cleanse the body using alfalfa, chamomile, cornsilk, and hyssop. According to their catalog (the Bible says, "Purge me with Hyssop and I shall be clean"). There are other herbal combinations for asthma, blood pressure, arthritis, colon cleansing, weight loss, isomnia, kidneys, eyes, lungs, acne, headaches, and allergies that can be ordered from their catalog.

Sex and the Mind

Just as the body affects the mind, so does the mind affect the body. No matter how alive and healthy one's body and dynamic one's sexual energy, fear, guilt, and antisexual programming from childhood miseducation can short-circuit this energy and turn it into psychosomatic symptoms. If such attitudes are extensive and deep-seated, help from a wholistic therapist is advisable. (See list at end of book.)

Suppressed feelings of anger and hurt are a major cause of diminished sexuality. For this reason, many couples find it necessary to provoke a "fight" in order to express and release these blocked emotions. Only then, in the process of "making up," are they able to feel and express their sexuality. But this is a tedious, tiresome, and stressful way of opening up which gradually damages tender loving feelings. It also fails to resolve the irrational conflicts that cause the hurt and anger.

There is a better way. I have successfully counseled many couples to use the Empathy Exercise I created to exorcize the negative emotions that create tension, block the loving flow of energy, and sabotage sexual pleasure. Each partner agrees to listen to the hurts and resentments of the other empathically (that is, without defending yourself or blaming the other for his or her feelings). Unless you can do this, you are incapable of caring for, respecting, and loving your partner. Love is an easy and empty word unless you can act in a loving way. Through honest sharing and communication in a caring way, the problems that create negativity can be solved and the way to warmth and pleasure cleared. (For a more detailed treatment of the empathy exercise, see Appendix II.)

Free Your Mind to Enhance Your Pleasure

A relaxed body and positive emotions go with a free mind, and vice versa. If you are harboring grudges, doubts, and negative thoughts about your partner, you can be sure your sexual freedom will suffer. Such thoughts and feelings can also be resolved with the empathy exercise (see page 305). If you or your partner are not capable of empathy or caring communication and are caught in the prison of the ego, your sexuality and your relationship will stagnate and wither away.

It is necessary to have a vital body, a free mind, and a warm heart—all three—to understand Henry Miller's words: "For whosoever lieth with a woman merely to gratify his sexual appetite has missed the supreme purpose and enjoyment of the act, which is to surrender one's heart and soul to the tender mercy of the beloved." The greatest aphrodisiac of all is love!

Chemicals, Sex, and Procreation

Researchers who do not work for the giant food processing companies see a connection between the proliferation of chemical additives in the artificial foods and drinks that fill our supermarkets and lessening of fertility in men. There are now some 5,000 chemical compounds that "enhance" our nourishment and that certainly interact with our bodies and with one another.

What does this have to do with sexual health and reproduction? The U.S. National Institute for Occupational Health and Safety reported that the average sperm count in American men has dropped to an all-time low in the last twenty-five years. Even when the low figure of a forty-million sperm count is taken as "normal" (a healthy count is

one-hundred million sperm per cubic centimeter of semen),
"the percentage of men with relatively low sperm counts had
almost doubled."[2]

To mitigate a tendency toward infertility, avoid all soft
drinks, junk foods, and snack and packaged foods that contain chemicals. Read labels. Buy fresh, natural and whole
foods — not only will you find yourself saving money, but
you will become more fresh, natural, and whole yourself.

You can also improve the functioning and increase the
energy flow to all the glands and organs of your body,
including those involved with your sexuality, by using the
reflexology techniques described in the following pages of
this book under the heading, Self Help with Reflexology.

The Syntonic Way to Improve
Your Sex Life

Physical Aspects

- Avoid sugar, fat, salt, nicotine, caffeine, and tap
  water that contains chlorine and fluoride.
- Get a second opinion from a nutritional physician
  regarding drugs you are taking that may be damaging your sexuality. Healthy alternatives can not only
  help you increase your sexual function, but also help
  you avoid iatrogenic (drug-induced) diseases.
- Have the same doctor check you for hypothyroid
  (low) imbalance if your libido is down, if you gain
  weight easily, if you are sensitive to cold, if you have
  dry skin, and if you lack zest for life.

---

[2] "Mean Sperm Counts in American Men Have Dropped," *Wall Street Journal*,
October 13, 1977.

- If your bowels do not function daily, have a check-up and ask if colonics and psysillium powder are indicated. A congested colon can affect the muscles involved in sexual functioning. A high-fiber and low-protein diet will also help.
- Avoid heavy eating and drinking before sex.
- Taking B vitamins from brewer's yeast, taking niacin before sex (it releases histamines, which are necessary in achieving orgasm), and zinc from pumpkin seeds, lecithin, and ginseng will also strengthen your sexual response.
- The herb ginkgo biloba and an aphrodisiac formula (No. 3) of several herbs, available from the Health Center for Better Living in Naples, Florida, have also proven to be helpful.
- By squeezing as if you are stopping urination, and then tightening and loosening these muscles slowly then quickly, you can free this area for the normal spasmodic function of orgasm for both women and men.

Emotional Aspects

- Your heart (i.e., your emotions) is at least as important as your hormones in sexuality, which in its true nature is love making. It is that personal element which combines tenderness and passion—yin and yang—and lifts sex from the mundane to the ecstatic.
- Often sex is misused to express anger toward one's partner. This dilutes the joy and meaning of love making and diminishes it to a merely physical release, devoid of deep satisfaction. If the free flow of loving energy is disturbed, do the empathy exercise (see

Appendix II) until the flow is restored. All the vitamins in the world cannot make up for an angry body or a cold heart.

Mental Aspects

- Hold one another closely, heart to heart, and, breathing slowly and deeply in unison, visualize your heart opening like a flower.
- If any fears come to mind that interfere with your freedom to open and love, share them with your partner. Gradually this will enable you to shift from the apprehensive (fight or flight) system to the secure, parasympathetic system. (See the Personality Chart.)
- As your mind is more clear, your trust will increase, your breathing will deepen, your body will relax, and your pleasure will heighten.

Spiritual Aspects

- Before you are ready to love another person, it is important to be at peace with the Higher Power. This means being in a Syntonic or whole state in harmony with the Life Force.
- The more you practice relaxing and feeling your body settling down and going with gravity ("not my will but Thine be done")—focusing your mind on slow breathing below your navel, and visualizing your *ki* or life force flowing outward toward the world—the more quickly you will be able to achieve this beautiful Syntonic state.
- If you first establish this state, you will never merely have sex—you will always experience it as making

love. Visualize it not as something you do but rather as something that happens through you. In surrendering to love and thereby losing oneself, one finds one's Self. Like meditation, in which one discovers "the peace that passeth understanding," loving surrender is a means to find Oneness with God.

Self-Help with Reflexology

I studied philosophy at Amherst College, comparative religion at Union Seminary, and premedicine and clinical and social psychology at Columbia University. I went on to postdoctoral work at the Psychiatric Institute, Bellevue Hospital, the Postgraduate Center for Psychotherapy, and the National Psychological Association for Psychoanalysis, where I became a senior analyst. But the most important education I received was in seeking to improve myself in different disciplines and kinds of therapy, with a variety of gurus and therapists. Gradually the four-dimensional approach—encompassing the body, mind, emotions, and spirit—evolved into Syntonic therapy.

Recently I took an intensive seminar with a scientist named Dr. Corwin West, who introduced me to further knowledge regarding the importance of avoiding the consumption of excessive animal protein and chemical additives. In Dr. West's concept, pain is caused by the blockage of lymph flow and circulation wherever this occurs in the body. I learned the importance of the nerve reflex centers of the feet in improving the functioning of every organ, gland, and cell. These reflexes have been used in the Orient for centuries to help the healing powers of the body. In Japan, a similar technique is called *shiatzu*, which means "finger pressure." Reflexology was brought to the attention of the healing professions in 1913 by William F. Fitzgerald, MD, who discovered that massaging certain reflex areas of the feet would help to improve the natural functioning of any part of the body connected with that particular zone.[3]

Reflexology appealed to me as an important addition to wholistic therapy for the following reasons: It is drugless and relatively painless; it helps the body function better in all its parts; it quickly and simply reveals (through the feet) the areas of the body that are toxic and congested before serious symptoms evolve; it motivates individuals to be more aware of their actual state of health; it enables them to take further responsibility for their own health; and it aids them to achieve greater vitality.

The root of mental health is in one's feet. When crippled by fear, we say that someone gets "cold feet." Similarly, "taking a stand" and "putting one's foot down" in an assertive manner (i.e., the ability to say no at the appropriate time) is a keynote of self-respect and maturity. Feet have further importance in total therapy. The toes, soles, heels, and ankles can reveal a great deal about your body. Chronic cases of illness which had not yielded to other methods of treatment have been healed by the surge of new energy resulting from reflexology.

If you avoid mental, emotional, and physical toxins by resolving destructive patterns of living, and at the same time help your body eliminate toxins and malfunctioning through reflexology, you will further your health and well-being. When teaching the reflex points while massaging the zones of someone's feet, I picture cosmic energy coming

---

[3] Mildred Carter, *Helping Yourself with Foot Reflexology*, Parker Publishing Company, Inc., West Nyack, New York.

through me, (energy directed by visualization) adding to the mechanical stimulation of the "reflex buttons." Following the reflexology charts on pages 92-94, I can locate areas of the body that are below par, whether or not the person is aware of them. Press each pont with a pencil eraser or the knuckle of your index finger. Pain will indicate a malfunction or toxicity in that area. I also use this means to motivate people to become more responsible about the violations they impose on their bodies, and to work more with their diet and other aspects of Syntonic therapy.

A daily self-massage of your reflex points will help you improve your health and well-being. For example, Mrs. X overcame a chronic problem through reflexology. She had suffered with a whiplash injury for six years, and as the wife of a physician she had undertaken numerous forms of treatment unsuccessfully. When I worked with the zone related to the right side of her neck and head (located on the top of her large right toe), the pain gradually eased and she moved her head freely for the first time in years.

Deep gland and organ malfunctioning, caused by a lifetime of tension and incorrect eating and living, require time and a total health regimen. Self-reflexology massage can help you improve other aspects of your emotional, mental, or spritual health. It will help you become relaxed, since tension in your feet involves every part of your being. It will also help you strengthen your endocrine glands and overcome addictions to drugs, overeating, alcohol, cigarettes, coffee, tea, or sugar.

Our endocrine glands utilize cosmic energy obtained through the food we eat and the air we breathe to create hormones, which influence all the activities of the body. Since every part of this many-trillioned cell universe is related, a deficiency of functioning of a single gland can

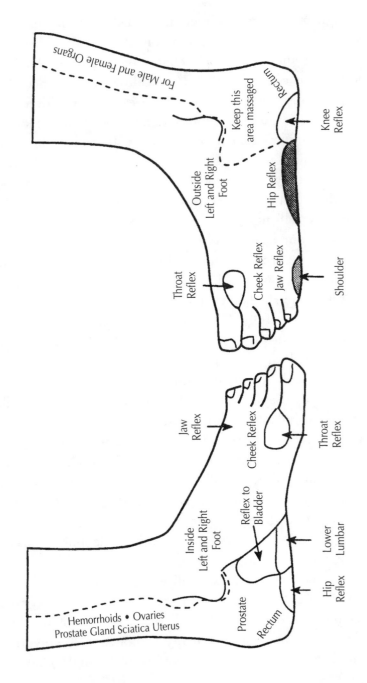

Head Cold Sinus and Hay Fever

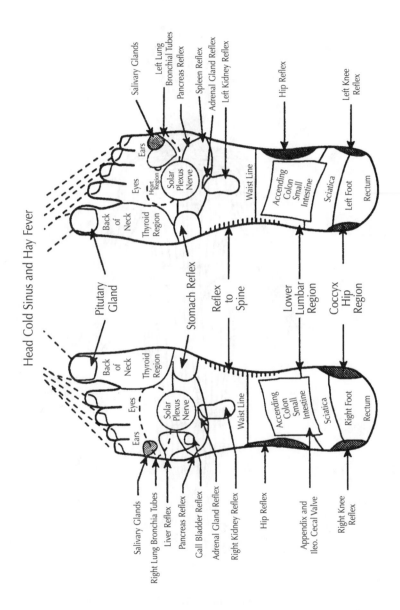

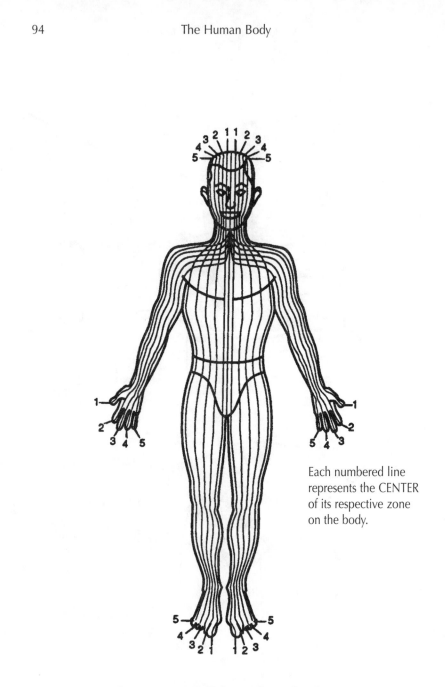

Each numbered line represents the CENTER of its respective zone on the body.

The Ten Zones Relating to the Reflexology Points on the Feet and Hands

throw our entire system out of homeostatic balance. When these "electrical generators" (called the seven *chakras* in esoteric philosophy) are not charged, fatigue can occur and cells can become stagnant and die, thus causing the body to suffer from toxemia or autointoxication. No wonder amazing things can happen when a tune-up is given through the foot reflexes!

An acquaintance recently called me in a very disturbed state, and understandably so. He had just been told that he needed an operation for an enlarged prostate. He came by for a therapy session, in the course of which I did some reflexology massage. The prostate reflexes on the inside of his ankles were indeed very sensitive, but in general his condition was somewhat toxemic with no other major areas of acute illness. Since his internist agreed, he decided to fast in order to help the healing powers of his body and perhaps to avoid surgery. A week of fasting and several weeks of self-reflexology, combined with intensive Syntonic therapy to help him release emotional and mental stress, strengthened the work of the "inner physician" and made surgery unnecessary.[4] His general health improved and he learned to take responsibility for his own health and well-being.

How Elizabeth Became Her Own Doctor

Another patient, Elizabeth, also had a rewarding experience with Syntonic therapy. Along with neurosis, she suffered from our old nemesis hypoglycemia, commonly known as low blood

---

[4] He also used zinc (50 gr. per day) and two herbal remedies—four capsules of corn silk and saw palmetto berries—per day. These can be ordered from the Health Center for Better Living in Naples, Florida.

sugar. This organic disturbance, in which the pancreas produces an excessive amount of insulin in the bloodstream, is often caused by many years of abusing one's body with white sugar, ice cream, desserts, cookies, etc. In this low blood sugar state, as we have seen, many typically neurotic symptoms occur (such as anxiety, claustrophobia, headaches, indigestion, lack of sexual drive, cold sweats, insomnia, crying spells, feelings of weakness and faintness, nightmares, and a sense that "something terrible is about to happen"). Something terrible is happening, since the glandular system is badly out of tune. Elizabeth was addicted to sweets, caffeine, and nicotine, a common syndrome for the disease. Each created a blood sugar low and a vicious circle of dependency. Her self-esteem was zero and suicide looked tempting. She was gaining weight and increasing toxemia in her body.

She was generally tense and anxious, and she depended on alcohol to sleep. Reflexology massage revealed not only extreme toxicity in the pancreas zone, but also in the adrenals, pituitary, kidneys, and uterus. As she gradually resolved emotional and mental patterns from a disturbed childhood in Syntonic therapy and changed to a natural whole food diet, she became less tense and toxic on all levels of her being. She learned to help herself with self hypnosis and meditation. Working with the foot reflexes herself between sessions, she was gradually able to achieve a better degree of syntony and harmony—physical, emotional, mental, and spiritual—than she had ever experienced. With a stabilized blood sugar level she no longer needed cigarettes and caffeine. Syntonic therapy saved Elizabeth's life.

Bill was also helped by the use of reflexology along with the other facets of Syntonic therapy. He had made considerable progress in overcoming his neurotic tendency to turn his anger on himself, instead of against the destructive patterns and images he carried within himself. He also made headway in changing old patterns of thinking that were crippling his positive forces and wasting his energies. His reflexes to the pituitary, adrenal, and kidneys were very sensitive to pressure on those points. But as these points were gradually massaged into healthier functioning, Bill made increasing progress toward personal responsibility and well-being. He was also more able to improve his diet and practice the release exercises and use of positive imagery, two facets of Syntonic therapy which will be explained later.

Daily massage of all reflex buttons on your feet is advisable. Since your kidneys are the organs which rid your body of many accumulated toxins, it is important to work very slowly and gently with the areas of the feet connected with them. Similarly, it is wise to make a slow transition to a healthy diet of whole grains, fruits, beans, vegetables (raw when possible), nuts, seeds, and seafood if desired, avoiding too rapid a release of toxins. Compare your nails and tongue before beginning this program, and two months afterward. Your nails will be smoother and stronger and your tongue will become pink and clean!

No Smoking, Please

No one can question the fact that cigarettes are "coffin nails." Statistics have shown that this habit robs *nine years* of the average smoker's life. The years prior to that premature death may also include diminished energy, hormonal imbalances, heart attacks, lung cancer, and the gradual suffocation of emphysema. The Surgeon General's Report early in 1980 warned that women now face the same epidemic of smoke-related diseases as men. The American Cancer Society reports that lung cancer, ranked eighth among cancer killers of women in 1961, has now become second only to breast cancer. And a study in Japan reports a twofold increase in lung cancer for nonsmoking women exposed to their husbands' smoking (the passive smoke danger, or secondary smoke).

These appalling facts have prompted many people to quit the habit, resulting in a slight decline in the number of smokers. Others have changed to low-tar and low-nicotine cigarettes. However, research at Columbia University suggests that smoking "safer" cigarettes may increase the danger, for two reasons. First, people tend to smoke more and inhale more deeply to get their "quota" of nicotine. Second, this increases the intake of "carbon monoxide, hydrogen cyanide and nitrogen oxides—gases implicated in cardivascular disease, respiratory problems, and fetal damage."[5]

There is additional evidence that cigarette smokers over age forty risk a 2,000 percent higher chance of developing lung cancer, and a higher incidence of sexual impotency due to smoking-related hormonal imbalances.

Reason would tell you to quit this deadly habit immediately, and some people do just that. However, some slip back into the habit, usually when stress increases in their life and they need to suck the substitute pacifier that harkens back to babyhood. Addictive persons—whether to smoking, food, alcohol, drugs, neurotic sex, or compulsive work—are driven by inner tension and anxiety to their misdirected and destructive behavior. If you are an addict, you know how cleverly the insecure child part of you can twist your reason and rationalize, "I'm going to quit soon," "Right now I need this crutch," "I don't want to live too long anyway." Insecure and immature people have a more difficult time giving up immediate pleasure in order to avoid later pain or to gain long-range satisfaction. Self-deception is a popular pastime. We often believe what we want to believe.

But don't condemn yourself for your weakness; rather,

---

[5] *The New York Times,* January 15, 1980.

become angry at the part of you, the insecure little child, that you allow to run your life. And remember, you are not alone in this struggle for maturity. Saint Augustine mentions in his classic *Confessions* that he prayed, "Make me good, Oh Lord, but not yet." Saint Paul said, "The good I would I do not; the evil I would not, that do I do." (Romans 7:15) Who among us can "cast the first stone"?

Different strategies for giving up bad habits seem to work for different people. If you are ready to save what is left of your health by the elimination of smoking—and wish to begin building your health—choose the suggestions from the following list that work for you. (These techniques can also be used to overcome other addictions.)

Eleven Ways to Kick the Habit

- The moment you have the impulse to reach for a cigarette,

1. Take a deep breath into your center, below your navel, and as you exhale let all tension and anxiety flow away from your body.

2. Picture your lungs full of tar and poisons as you inhale; and picture them being cleansed as you exhale.

3. Do something to divert your attention from cigarettes. Chew a carrot or sugarless gum; do a few pushups or situps; put a few cushions on the floor and "put your foot down" assertively, with a feeling of taking charge rather than being weak and helpless. Or lie down and kick out your legs with the idea in mind of "kicking the habit." Yell into a pillow as loudly as you can, "I'm tired of ruining

my health," using positive anger to overcome your dependency.

4. Carry a pad with you and each time before you take a cigarette write, "Do I really want to take years off my life and hasten a horrible death?"

5. Carry with you pictures of lungs ravaged by cancer and emphysema. Your local chapter of the American Cancer Society will furnish you with them. Promise yourself that you will look at this picture before you light each cigarette. Also keep another such picture in full view in your home.

6. Release the tension that underlies the impulse to smoke by doing several head rolls. Bring your shoulders to your ears as you inhale, and drop and relax them as you exhale.

7. Read all you can about the insidious effects of smoking on billions of cells in your body.

8. Use a holder with a filter, if you find that you are delaying your final decision. Examine the filter each day for contents that would have been futher poisoning your body. Smell and taste this residue and then carefully wash out your mouth.

9. Several times a day, take a minute to sit quietly, breathe gently into the center of your body, and feel your weight going with gravity. As your mind becomes more quiet and peaceful, say to yourself, "I value my body and my health; cigarettes have no place in my life."

10. Many people stop smoking and substitute overeating and drinking to deal with their underlying anxiety and tension. To avoid becoming overweight, they often return to smoking as the "lesser" of the two evils. This is an ideal time to change from the

"killer" low-fiber, high-fat, and refined food diet to the healthy, high-energy, and high-fiber diet of whole grains, vegetables, and fruits. Since this low-fat diet is the natural diet for humans, you will gradually and inevitably reach your proper weight this way. My patients who give up sweets and junk food find they no longer have sugar "lows" and no longer "need" the nicotine boost!

11. Daily exercise and stretching, along with sports, when possible, or two miles of brisk walking will help to eliminate tension, blocked energy, and depression. The techniques described in the following chapters to release negative emotions and build positive feelings, along with changing your thinking patterns and strengthening your connection with the Life Force, will further improve your *joie de vivre*. The greater your self-esteem and happiness, the less you will need smoking or any other self-destructive habit.

For Marijuana Smokers

Smoking marijuana can have beneficial effects if you are a cancer victim and wish to reduce nausea caused by anti-cancer drugs. Otherwise, according to researchers, marijuana is a major and serious public health hazard. Along with subjecting the body to tar products and carbon monoxide, marijuana disturbs the sleep level of the user, leads to fatigue, causes hormonal changes in the body that have a negative effect on potency and the male and female reproductive systems.[6]

---

[6] Harvard Medical School Letter, Volume 4, Number 5.

For patients in therapy, marijuana smoking tends to undermine motivation to change and increase the tendency to withdraw from reality into fantasy. I have found that it also increases the anxiety and paranoid tendencies of more disturbed patients.

A recent survey of high school seniors indicates that one in ten smoke marijuana, double the number of five years ago.[7] I believe that this is a result of inadequate health education, faulty nutrition (remember the symptoms of hypoglycemia?), and the deplorable lack of courses in schools to help students deal with their emotional conflicts, tensions, and anxieties. Like all addicts they use an "escape" that only compounds their problems. (see Appendix IV.)

The same anticigarette techniques cited earlier, along with an overall change to a health-building, wholistic lifestyle, can be used to overcome the marijuana habit.

Using Kinesiology to Improve Your Health

Kinesiology is the study of movement and muscle function. It is possible to test the effect of various foods, materials, and sounds on your whole body by testing the effects they may have on your muscular responses; that is a strengthening or weakening effect.

Your energy is diminished by negative thoughts, cigarette smoke, poor-quality foods, and plastic materials since everything has a vibratory rate. I have taught many people to use this muscle-testing technique to help themselves and others.

---

[7] *The New York Times,* January 17, 1980.

To test the effect of tobacco on your Life Force, for example, try this experiment. Stand about two feet away from another person, face to face. Hold your left arm straight out from your body. Have your tester place his or her left hand on your shoulder, and firmly push down on your left fist while you try to keep it up. See illustration on page 104. If you feel very weak, thump on your thymus gland in your upper chest (the way gorillas do when they become excited). Then try again. Next put a cigarette in your mouth and repeat the test. You can also test the effect of cigarettes by holding a pack in your hand against your navel. Does your Life Force increase or decrease? Is your arm weaker or stronger?

Try this same test with sugar, milk, natural honey, animal fat, whole wheat, white bread, and salt, etc. You can also test the effect of different sounds and music on your life energy. This technique fits beautifully into a wholistic self-improvement program. It offers proof that rock music, junk and refined foods, plastic fabrics, and cigarettes seriously weaken the Life Force in your body and pave the way toward disease and premature death.

But test these things for yourself as a part of the responsibility you have assumed to be your own doctor. If Mozart, whole foods, natural cotton or wool clothing, and healthy lungs put bounce in your step and a sparkle in your eyes, you'll be far ahead of most people who walk with a heavy step and forget how wonderful it is to be alive—really and truly alive.

Additionally, you can test vitamins, medications, and foods or supplements to which you may be allergic. Some children and adults have particular allergies to substances such as wheat, milk, chocolate, and food additives and colorings, which may cause intense emotional and psychological symptoms. You can also test for yourself the difference

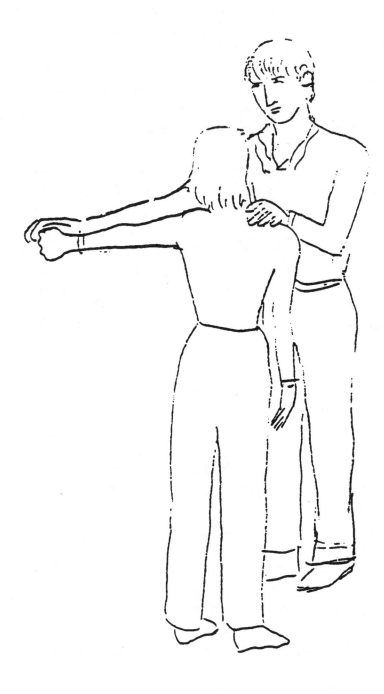

between the effect on your Life Force of organic foods and foods which have been sprayed with insecticides. Compare regular and herb tea, and find out the effect of chemical sweeteners on your precious Life Force. Test different foods to determine whether you are best suited to being vegetarian.

The Prudent Low-Fat Health and Longevity Diet

Your diet for optimal health should be a high fiber diet of whole natural foods free of poisons and pesticides: brown rice, whole grains, beans of all varieties, sunflower and sprouted alfalfa seeds, raw or lightly steamed vegetables, and fruits (unless you are hypoglycemic) in their natural state. Breads should be made with stone ground flour without sugar or salt; seasonings with natural soy sauce (tamari), garlic, kelp and herbs. Salad dressings should be made with apple cider vinegar, low fat yogurt and cold pressed oils. Nuts without salt, and dried fruits without sulphur may be used in moderation along with seafood and free range fowl if appropriate.

Drinks: pure water (best if filtered or steam distilled), herb teas such as linden, alfalfa, rose hips and green tea. Avoid coffee, or use a kind decaffeinated by a natural process, without chemicals. Dark and natural honey may be used in moderation if you do not have blood sugar problems.

Ways to Improve Your Health and Vitality

- Plan time for the suggested physical exercises at the start of your day—to tune up every part of your body.

- Perform exercises without clothing so your whole body can breathe.
- After exercises, when breathing is fuller and more complete, do the relaxation and centering exercises.
- On particularly tense and anxious days, use the emotional release techniques described in the next section, before the centering and positive imagery techniques.
- Do the brisk body rub before bathing.
- Do the alimentary massage to help your intestines perform their important eliminative work.
- Remember your center and your breathing at all times, for greater security and aliveness.
- If you lose sleep one night, make up for it the next.
- Take a few minutes of your lunch hour to center and get back in tune with the Cosmic Flow; then enjoy a healthy lunch.
- When possible, help your digestion and assimilation with proper food combining, as described in the chart on page 51.
- If you or a member of your family has allergies, try the elimination diet or muscle testing.
- To improve sexual vigor, total self-improvement is necessary along with the exercises, breathing, and the use of vitamin, mineral, and herbal supplements. The empathy exercise will help resolve emotional blockages that negate sexual love.
- Give yourself a daily five-minute reflexology massage.
- Use my techniques to quit smoking. If necessary, obtain hypnosis.

An Affirmation for Non-Smoking to Save Your Life

The thought of poisoning my lungs is disgusting.

I want clean blood flowing through my body.

I respect the gift of the trillions of cells that comprise my Self.

I glory in the miracle of life.

My center is below my navel where I breathe deeply.

The more I focus on my center the more whole I become.

The more I unify my mind and body the stronger I am.

Being strong I no longer need this poisonous crutch.

I feel more and more free of this addiction.

I find strength in the Life Force itself.

I am grateful for the priceless gift of health.

I love myself as a child of God.

I no longer pollute "the temple of the Spirit", my body.

My self-esteem comes from the Higher Power.

Realizing my true worth, I am a non-smoker.

Every breath is a priceless gift that connects me to God.

I visualize myself free in body, emotions, mind, and Spirit.

Each day I grow in gratitude, health, and happiness.

Please make a tape of this for yourself, adding your own special affirmation from your heart and mind. Then focus on one point as you sit comfortably in an easy chair, count to five, and at the five count close your eyes and go within to your center below your navel. Then play your tape while you are in this deep receptive state at least once a day. At the end melt into the Silence for several minutes; then come back to the finite world rejuvenated and renewed! Then, as the masters taught, you will happily be "in the world but not of it."

The Human Emotions

Hell is the condition of those
who cannot love.

—DOSTOYEVSKY
THE BROTHERS KARAMAZOV

Love casts out fear.

—THE BIBLE
I JOHN 4:18

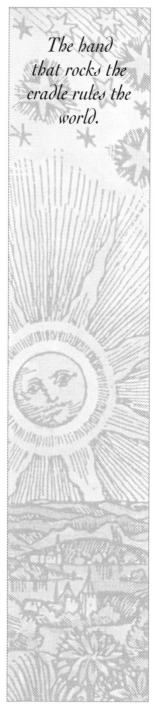

The hand that rocks the cradle rules the world.

FIVE

The Roots of Emotional Disease

Blocked versus Flowing Emotions

Since neurotic individuals have learned to develop tension (which can be imagined as a sort of muscular armor) as protection from outer hurt and as a way of repressing forbidden inner feelings, their ability to emote (literally, "to move out") is damaged. Healthy people are concerned with living, growing, risking, and fulfillment. They have the courage and vitality to "take arms against a sea of

111

troubles" if they arise. On the contrary, neurotic people will tend to suffer—and either passively settle for safety or react irrationally or violently. Humans' autonomic nervous makeup—the sympathetic and parasympathetic—is delicately balanced between anxiety and security, fear and trust, hate and love. When this system is negatively conditioned in the earliest formative years, humans lean toward anxiety, tension, and the tendency to project and provoke dangers that do not exist.

Thus, neurotic people are never emotionally free, for chronic anxiety (generalized fear) triggers their primitive inclination to withdraw, to fight, or to submit. Consciously or unconsciously, neurotic people are always torn by these conflicting drives. Instead of flowing pleasurably, the stream of their life is dammed up within. Sometimes this stream builds up and breaks the dam. The chronic emergency reaction results in self-defeating feelings of depression, inferiority, worthlessness, and a variety of psychosomatic symptoms—along with the compulsion to find masochistic "solutions" in, for example, alcoholism, drug addiction, obsessive work, compulsive sex, or escape into fantasy. When neurotic individuals learn to act out their tension and hostility—to break the dam, as it were—the result is antisocial, sadistic, and violent behavior.

Robbed of the human birthright, which is the feeling of love and well-being—"I am, I am of value, I am part of life, and life is good"—disturbed and anxious people question their self-worth, their identity, and they feel alienated from life. A deep meaninglessness prevails: "Who am I?" "I have no value," and "What is the point of life?" Sometimes this is hidden beneath grandiosity. It is written in Ecclesiastes: "All is vanity and vexation of spirit." Shakespeare also illustrated this attitude: "We strut and fret our brief hour on the stage, and then are heard no more." And Thoreau saw most of humanity as living lives of "quiet desperation."

The myth of the Garden of Eden in the Bible suggests that humans' ability to think, to reflect, to conceptualize, and to transcend nature separated them from the instinctual and uncomplicated life of the animal world. Humans developed the "freedom" to violate the order of nature — the "cardinal sin" of pride in the Judeo-Christian tradition, or "hubris" in Greek religion. The human infant is totally dependent far longer than any other species, and accordingly is more vulnerable to environmental influences. This would suggest that miseducation and not human perversity is the root of emotional disease. The British psychoanalyst Anthony Storr, who has defined humans as "the paranoid primate," would agree with my diagnosis. He also sees humans' destructive and cruel tendencies as stemming from the way in which we rear our infants, suggesting that "cultures which maintain a closer contact between mother and infant for a longer period may reduce this paranoid tendency."

A society like ours, in which cases of child abuse and wife beating number in the millions each year, needs radical changes from birth on to preserve the basic goodness in human nature.

Two Primitive Societies and One Advanced Society

It is fascinating to note that "primitive" peoples also experience the gamut of emotions. Margaret Mead's magnificent cross-cultural studies of South Sea societies show that among adults in societies where infants are nursed lovingly, and where children are treated with affection and respect, positive emotions predominate.[1] "The Samoan mother nurses her child generously . . . he is given food, consoled, carried about . . . he is fed when he is hungry, carried when he is tired, allowed to sleep when he wills." Mead describes the Samoans as "peaceful and constructive as a people," who "plant and reap, fish and build, feast and dance, in a world where no one is hurried . . . and life is harmonious and unintense." She describes the love between parents and children and notes that "the Samoan adult sex adjustment may be said to be one of the smoothest in the world." This society clearly demonstrates the relationship between emotional health in infancy and childhood and mature and happy adulthood. More emotionally secure and flexible, "the Samoans have made one of the most effective adjustments to the impact of Western civilization of any known people."

In contrast to the emotionally peaceful, loving, and joyful Samoans, Mead describes another society, the cannibal Mundugumor, as a "restive people who prey upon the miserable, underfed bush people, devote their time to quarreling and head hunting and have developed a form of social organization in which every man's hand is against every other man." Furthermore, "the women detest bearing and rearing children, and provide most of the food, leaving the men free to plot and fight." In contrast to the Samoans and most significant for the destructive emotional characteristics and behavior of this group, "pregnancy and nursing are hated and avoided if possible."

If an alien anthropologist from some rational, healthy, and civilized planet were to visit us, he or she would describe the peoples of the industrial nations of Earth as follows:

---

[1] Margaret Mead, Male and Female, William Morrow and Co. Pub., 1949.

In contrast to the emotionally peaceful, loving, and joyful Samoans, the people of the industrial nations are a restive people who pray on Sunday, and prey the rest of the week on the miserable, underfed people in their own and weaker countries. Often they make war to divert attention from unrest and injustice; and to relieve their sense of worthlessness they blindly follow their psychopathic leaders in the name of patriotism. Many devote their time to quarrelling and punishing their troublesome children, all of whom suffer from frustrated infancies, or to hunting for other groups or minorities that they can scapegoat.

They have developed a form of social organization in which every person's hand is against every other person, and the police cannot control rampant crime from the lowest to the highest levels of society, or even among their own forces. More and more women, feeling inadequate from their own infancy, shrink from bearing and rearing children and find work their liberation, leaving the men to plot and prepare for greater wars in the name of freedom, justice, and lasting peace. In the majority of women, due to the effects of their own deprived infancies, pregnancy and nursing are hated and avoided if possible. They nurse by the ingenious invention of artificial and destructive formulas, plastic bottles, and rubber nipples.

Infants are isolated in sterile maternity wards and suffer from premature weaning, all under the direction of learned specialists called pediatricians. Meanwhile, their social scientists decry what they call The Age of Alienation and the myriad symptoms which accompany this unnatural condition. One wonders if they see any relationship between this phenomenon and the fact that they, alone among the earthly mammals, initiate their offspring in pain, frustration, tension, and anxiety from earliest infancy.

Restoring Healthy Loving Contact to Your Life

There are hopeful signs, however, in the growth of natural childbirth, the natural and nonviolent birthing techniques of Lamaze and Leboyer, and the increasing realization that when hospital personnel intrude on the relationship between the newborn and its mother, both are harmed. Many hospitals separate mothers and newborns for the first several days of life. Drs. Klaus and Kennel, in their book *Maternal-Infant Bonding*,[2] point out that immediate close contact is crucial to the well-being of newborn and mother and basic to the formation of a deep and lasting relationship between them. They point out that infants deprived of such contact "fail to thrive, grow, gain weight, and develop naturally."

After my book *Understanding Homosexuality* was published by Macmillan and circulated throughout the world, I worked with many sincere men from fifteen different countries who wanted to become heterosexual. Many achieved their goal, but every one had had a fractured love bond with their mothers, and developed a "fear bond" which undermined sexual feelings toward women. Lacking loving energy contact, mothers often think of their babies as belonging to someone else, and children with such a threatened personality foundation often think that their "real" parents are other than the ones they have. They found that early-contact mothers gave more love to their babies, nursed longer and more easily, and their babies in turn cried

---

[2] Marshall Klaus and John Kennel, *Maternal Infant Bonding*, C.B. Mosby Co., St. Louis, Mo., 1976.

less and smiled and laughed more, evincing signs of happiness and relaxation. A study in Sweden found that immediate contact between mother and infant after birth resulted in fewer problems and richer closeness later on, as we saw above in Dr. LeBoyer's studies.

Attitudes and personality patterns are formed earlier in development than is generally realized. One can believe a Yale University researcher who said, "It [formation of attitudes and personality patterns] is more or less over by the age of three." The implications of these facts for overall human health are staggering. Even pre-birth experiences have major effects on personality development.[3]

For those of us who did not have the benefit of a natural birth and a happy infancy; our potential for love and joy is limited accordingly. Undoing the fears and tensions rooted in our muscles, nerve circuits, and emotional conditioning is not an easy challenge and demands a total program of self-reeducation, which Syntonics is designed to help you accomplish.

Points to Remember Regarding the Emotional Problems That Plague our Society

- Our biological makeup makes us vulnerable to negative emotional conditioning.
- This learning takes place from birth onward, and in some instances from prenatal traumatic experiences.
- Negative feelings can turn against oneself and, in many instances, against others as well.

---

[3] Thomas Verney, M.D., *The Secret Life of The Unborn Child*, Delta Pub., N.Y., 1981.

- The core of human beings is creative and loving.
- Anthropological studies reveal the conditions that nurture or damage and distort the creative nature of humans.
- There is increasing awareness of the importance of natural, nonviolent childbirth, nursing, and infant-mother bonding.
- Wholistic Syntonic therapy and self-education offer the opportunity for emotional growth and improvement.
- Spread the word about the benefits of nonviolent childbirth and the importance of nursing for mother and infant whenever possible.
- Use all facets of Syntonics—physical, emotional, mental, and spiritual—to help yourself move toward your healthy Self on the Personality Chart. (p. xxvii). Specific techniques will be outlined in the following pages.
- Practice the Empathy Exercise (p. 305) to create a more positive relationship with people close to you.
- Spread the word about the way to a happy family, as described in Appendix I

SIX

Free Yourself from Chronic Fear and Anxiety

My clinical experience has shown that it is far easier to improve your emotional health and balance if you have a healthy body free from toxemia and enervation.

Avoiding stress and building emotional health depend on a whole way of life in balance with nature. Such a health revolution must be built upon a healthy body, sound nutrition, and a positive lifestyle.

There are also emotional toxins from faulty childhood conditioning

119

(see the Personality Chart) that produce *chronic* underlying fear or anxiety. This malady must not be confused with realistic fear, which is a protective and life-sustaining reaction to actual outer danger. Without the instantaneous reaction of fear to an actual threat, life would not be able to continue. No species could have survived what Charles Darwin called "the quiet and dreadful war" that occurs around us (i.e., there could not be survival of the fittest) without a mechanism for flight or fight.

But when this mechanism of fear is engaged chronically, adrenalin constantly infuses the bloodstream and we are caught in an endless state of tension wherein all natural and pleasurable functions of the organism are suspended or even crippled. Under this stress, the basic functions of life are strained—the appetite is unbalanced, breathing is inhibited, digestion is impeded, respiration is hindered, glandular processes are disturbed, blood pressure is increased, organ functioning is impaired, elimination is blocked, heartbeat is accelerated, sexuality is undermined, and hostility and tension are cultivated.

Wilhelm Reich described this condition as[1] "chronic sympatheticatonia," or the constant domination of the organism by the sympathetic nervous system, the function which is involved with survival reactions. In contrast, the secure organism enjoys a relaxed and pleasurable state of syntony and well-being, regulated by the parasympathetic system. After realistic danger has passed, the emotionally healthy person is free to return to this inner state of emotional harmony. All addictions, with their damaging effects on body, mind, and spirit, stem from this chronic state of anxiety that

---

[1] Wilhelm Reich, *The Function of the Orgasm*, Orgone Institute Press., N.Y., 1948.

is so common in our society. Furthermore, 85 percent of all illness is stress related according to many doctors. Most of us have lost that healthy state of self, indicated at the center of the Personality Chart. We may have glimpses of it, like rays of sunlight filtering through clouds—but *only* glimpses. The goal of Syntonics reeducation is therefore to rediscover, maintain, and strengthen one's authentic Self.

Underneath the facades with which most people attempt to deceive themselves and others, the anxious inner child is still painfully imprisoned. This is just as true for the average person as it is for executives, writers, physicians, and psychoanalysts—for monetary or intellectual power and academic achievement do not engender emotional maturity. The mass disease of loneliness is a general symptom of this condition, driving the helpless individual to drink or to engage in other futile and self-destructive attempts to escape inner fears and terrors. Pascal had a deep insight into this inner desperation: "Most of man's difficulties stem from the fact that he cannot spend ten minutes quietly with himself in a room alone."

One of my patients, Silas, was a typical example of this syndrome. The victim of disturbed and cruel parents who were themselves victims of *their* parents, Silas repeatedly and blindly acted out his childhood pattern of running away in panic. He had often done this as a child until his father chained him up to "teach him a lesson." As an adult, he repeated this pattern with his wife and family, going away whenever inner tensions built up to the point that he felt that he might do violence against his wife and family. (At times he would project these violent urges onto his wife and feared that she would kill him in his sleep.) After running in panic for a while, Silas would repeatedly feel guilty at leaving his wife and family and, afraid of being alone, would return to repeat the same pattern. Unfortunately, he did the same thing in therapy. Unable to face the panic, rage, and helplessness of the inner child, he ran from the very help he needed desperately.

The Human Energy Crisis

Chronic fear or anxiety drives one to insoluble and painful conflicts. One is torn between the impulse to attack, to remove the apparent threat to one's life; to flee and save oneself; or to submit and placate the outer enemy.

One mode of neurotic behavior appears and sometimes switches to another, either instantaneously or gradually. But underneath, these conflicting behaviors are part of humankind's biological reaction to fear. This distortion of the emergency reaction is the greatest energy crisis of our planet, for it short-circuits the potentially flowing and creative energy of billions of miseducated human beings into destructive channels: illness, crime, violence, and war. They, in turn, pass this on to the next generation.

The formula can be described as follows: anxiety = energy + conflicts + tension. Energy becomes blocked by inner conflicts and muscular tension. Just as blocked energy on a physical level (e.g., a sprained ankle or a stomach spasm) results in physical pain, blocked emotional energy results in emotional pain. One becomes emotionally toxic, caught between attacking, running, or submitting—between anger, fear, or hopelessness. All of one's health, digestion, and rationality become undermined. The same thing would happen to a car if the driver simultaneously pressed the accelerator, pushed on the brake, and twisted the steering wheel in all directions.

A healthy emotional state is one in which there is a basic feeling of well-being and security. This can be described as follows: happiness = vitality + love + positive assertion. One is free of old conditioning; and instead of acting out past patterns of survival behavior, one is free to act in present reality in a clear and positive manner. No longer fearfully dependent on others or trapped in the outmoded behaviors of the inner child, one lets one's energies flow in a body that is free of unnatural tension. In this state, one can risk, grow, and enjoy the gift of every breath and moment of being.

Regain Your Real Self

This is not to say that life does not present the healthy person with problems. But problems become challenges and opportunities for further growth. There will also be sorrow, tears, realistic fears, and moments requiring assertiveness. But the basic feeling is that life is good, and feelings of faith, hope, and love (the fruits of the Holy Spirit) are dominant. Physically and emotionally healthy people are naturally real, open, positive, and life affirming. They can accept the loss of a loved one or a job without depression or despair. They are strong enough to admit that they can be hurt or disappointed and go on from there. Without wasting energy on defenses and deceit or pretensions to perfection, they have genuine strength and courage.

Nor does the truly vital person fear criticism or rejection by others, or give other people the power to decide his or her own value. We are brought up with the nonsense that we are only of value if we perform well. A good performance is rewarded with, "You're a good girl [or a good boy]." We have been brainwashed into feeling that we are not a valuable part of creation unless we earn such value. Only societies that give infants and children healthy physical and emotional nourishment provide the conditions for establishing a society of freedom through self-assertion and justice, in which the needs and rights of others are also important. The attitude of the emotionally free person is "If I am not for myself, who will be? If I am not for others, what am I?"

For many years I suffered from this type of fear and blocked energy. I had been able to write philosophy papers for deadlines in the process of gaining degrees from Amherst College, papers in comparative religion at Union Theological Seminary, and papers in clinical psychology at Columbia University. But when it came to writing for myself, I had what is known as writer's block. My energy was indeed blocked by fear—the fear of expressing my ideas, feelings, and experiences. My pattern, like the conditioning of most people who were raised in authoritarian homes and schools, was to be careful and safe, and thus avoid mother's hurt or father's anger.

This blocking of energy flow through fear—along with the toxemia and tension described in earlier chapters—kept me from what is now one of the joys of my life. Now I can speak freely and write spontaneously. I enjoy the pleasure of expressing the things I feel, think, value, and believe. How? By Syntonics—the very same process of freeing my body, emotions, mind, and spirit that is described in these pages. Now I look forward to writing, enjoy the flow of energy, and am ready to play tennis or go dancing after six hours at my typewriter, or with patients.

What can one do for oneself to improve emotional health? Are there specific emotional exercises as tangible as the physical program outlined earlier? There are indeed. But first let us explore the key to emotional change and growth—how you can use in a productive way the anger that always accompanies fear and sadness, whether it is on the surface or hidden underneath.

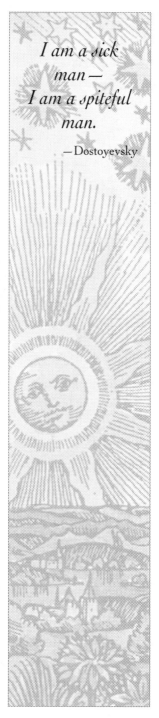

I am a sick man — I am a spiteful man.

—Dostoyevsky

SEVEN

The Power of Positive Anger

Of the three negative emotions in the "unholy trinity" of fear, hopelessness, and anger, only anger has a potentially outgoing force. I say *potentially* because anger is often repressed and buried through guilt and fear, muscular tension, and armoring. All guilt, in my view, is not neurotic or destructive. But neurotic guilt is anger turned destructively upon oneself and is nonproductive. It wastes energy, creates feelings of worthlessness, and reactivates the

125

inner "bad child" that most of us carry over from early life.

This kind of self-hurting is masochistic and wasteful of energy that could otherwise be used for growth. In my personal struggle, I used to be angry at myself for not writing and for becoming blocked by fear; I put myself down for not being productive. This would lead to envy of colleagues who were writing books. And this constant comparison of myself to others was another source of feeling guilty, for a decent person doesn't resent the successes of friends or acquaintances. I know what the French novelist Anatole France meant when he confessed, "I get secret pleasure from the misfortunes of my friends."

But somewhere I also knew that this was not my true Self. Rather, it was myself as a frightened child being undermined by my inner angry parent, who was telling me, "You're no good if you don't produce and write!" Then I would spite myself (the inner parent part of me) and not write and feel guilty again. Sometimes I became irritable and frustrated and took my tension out on others. That led to more destructive guilt at being a "difficult husband," "bad father," or "rotten friend."

Gradually it dawned on me that I *should* feel guilty about this behavior. But instead of making it worse by turning my anger on myself and others, I decided to turn it on the inner enemy—namely, my fear—and the inner negative parental images I was carrying around and "spiting" by hurting myself. With myself and the patients with whom I was working, this became the key to dynamic change. No matter what our past, blaming others or blaming ourselves is a clever cop-out. It keeps us spinning our wheels, getting nowhere, and settling for the secondary satisfaction of self-pity, martyrdom, and bolstering our little egos by putting others down.

Healthy Guilt

Once I accepted that I alone was the architect of my own tension, neurotic guilt, and frustration, I accepted as healthy my feeling of guilt; that I was not fulfilling my potential as a person and giving back to life at least a part of what life had so generously given me. Healthy guilt means to challenge one's pettiness, fear, spite, and the endless little games of one's "inner devil," one's egoistic negative inner child.

I had discovered a constructive target for my anger and for the power in myself and my patients; I call this power the "rage to live." Instead of taking my anger out through self-blame, spite, perfectionistic criticism, and irritability, I turned it on my inner enemies—those parts of me that prevented me from being free and productive. I could then, in Shakespeare's words, "take arms against a sea of troubles and, by opposing, end them!"

Just as fire can be used for good or ill, the power of anger can be used as a positive or destructive force. Just as the healthy forces in society destroy the ghettos and build communities where human beings can live decently, one must destroy the inner areas of waste and stagnation and build anew. As I overcame fear of my own rage and learned to use it constructively, I found that this was the key to dynamic emotional growth—not just arid intellectual insight. No longer afraid of my rage to live, I became able to help others discover, accept, and utilize constructively the anger they had locked up in tense bodies or had displaced on others.

The Background of Syntonic Therapy

In Syntonic therapy, I no longer worked exclusively with words as I had for a number of years, as a trained psychoanalyst. The word *psychoanalyst* indicates a preoccupation with the psyche or mind, which is only the tip of the iceberg and excludes far greater dimensions of the human being. Freud realized the shortcomings of his technique and stated that "from time to time I visualize a second part to the method of treatment; liberating patients' feelings as well as their ideas—as if this were quite indispensable."[1]

Since patients' words are so often out of touch with their feelings, I encourage them to make spontaneous sounds and movements in order to thaw out frozen energies that have been locked up in pain, depression, and tension. Deeper respiration is mobilized and quickly triggers emotions that have been buried or repressed. Memories then come into awareness in an emotionally alive manner, rather than being talked about in an abstract, merely verbal fashion.[2]

Freud was an iconoclast to the established ideas of his day. In a time of Victorian prudery, he saw that sexuality— beginning in infancy—was a fundamental fact of life. He understood the depths of human nature: the potential for the demonic, as well as the creative. Moreover, Freud realized that the mind is only one part of humans, and that humans' emotional life underlies their rationality, as the Bible expresses: "Out of the heart are the issues of life." Freud realized—through explorations with hypnosis and with his psychoanalytic method of free association—that the effect of past experiences exists in the present, but beyond the patient's awareness.

---

[1] Letter to his friend, Dr. Fliess, 1897.

[2] R. Kronemeyer, Syntonic Therapy: A Total Approach to the Treatment of Mental and Emotional Disturbances, *Psychotherapy: Theory, Research and Practice.* Volume 14. No. 1, Fall 1977.

Another aspect of Freud's contribution was his open mind to discovery. As a true scientist, Freud was not limited by a need to hold onto a closed system, which is a characteristic of his followers even today. The story goes that once Freud was asked, after a lecture, why a recent statement of his contradicted something he had written earlier. Freud in amusement replied, "I am not a Freudian."

I believe that the developments in the total therapy I practice are in accord with this spirit. In the history of humanity's quest for greater understanding through the scientific method of questioning and experimentation, the heresy of today often becomes the orthodoxy of tomorrow. Freud developed a new technique. But many people, in Freud's day as now, cannot be reached by verbal methods alone. Freud stressed the necessity of catharsis—expressing blocked emotions and freeing the bound-up energies of the organism. This is like freeing a stream that becomes dammed up and stagnant. And in catharsis, too, Freud sensed the need for working with more than the mind. He also wrote in a letter to his friend Dr. Fliess, "Some day psychoanalysis will be put on a biological foundation."

After Freud, another great iconoclast, Wilhelm Reich, made great contributions which to some extent fulfilled Freud's prediction. By focusing on the "character armor"— the way in which the person denies or guards against his or her true emotions—he helped patients challenge rather than maintain their ways of defense, which were necessary in childhood but in adulthood are part of their self-imprisonment (see defenses in the Personality Chart). Reich's view of the neurotic process involved the tensions, muscular attitudes, and mannerisms that are part of every person. He called this the "muscular armor," and this describes exactly what chronic tensions are—ways of holding one's body, developed from childhood for self-protection.

Notice on the Personality Chart that as we experience destructive home and school environments, we gradually lose touch with our undisturbed Self. Our negative emotions often become chronic, our defenses become hardened, and our muscular rigidity increases.

I was fortunate to have had therapy and training with Reich when I was a doctoral student. After a year of nondirective therapy with a passive therapist, I was still caught in anxiety, buried sadness, and rage, which had been carried over from the conflicts and tensions of my past. Under Reich's training, I found what I had been seeking. I was no longer able to sit passively and talk about myself despite the frightening volcano which churned within. Reich revealed to me my characteristic way of denying and binding the very emotions which I subconsciously knew had to be expressed. He indicated my "neurotic calm" manner in which I was blocking myself from freedom, and he encouraged me to breathe rather than hold my breath in a constant attempt to control my feelings, and express my sadness and rage.

Thus, Reich's revolutionary methods were a great advance over Freud's verbal technique of free association, in which the patient tries through words alone to become free—only to become trapped in the very web from which he or she was trying to escape. Reich, standing on Freud's shoulders, saw farther and went beyond the accepted methods of his day. In doing so, he inspired many of us to try new and more total methods of helping troubled people regain their Syntony and health.

One change in my practice that occurred after studying with Reich was in the doctor-patient relationship. Reich had the medical approach: Like a surgeon who was going to operate whether you liked it or not, Reich was going to cure your neurosis. But this insistence only increases the patient's tendency to resist change. We all tend to keep our old ways unless we realize the actual price we are paying for them. The frightened child within us will try to maintain these defenses when the doctor tries to take them away. He or she will spite the doctor as a parent substitute and stay "safely neurotic." This resistance is strong, for it is composed of all the ways we have developed to protect ourselves from painful emotions and punishment. But as the therapist attacks the "character armor" and "muscular armor," most patients are not strong enough to handle their fear and anger that results in relation to the doctor.

This happened to me with Reich. He was a powerful, unpredictable, and explosively expressive man. Like many creative geniuses, he was not emotionally balanced and mature. He could blow hot and cold, and he possessed a rage that could ignite very easily. Therapy was something he did "to" the patient. Though he helped me release some of the tension connected with buried sadness, in this authoritarian atmosphere I was not able to work with my inner rage and grow toward healthy self-assertion.

Liberate Yourself With Syntonic Therapy

Gradually I realized that a domineering therapist is just as counterproductive as a passive one. In Syntonic therapy, I make it clear to my clients that I cannot cure them. Rather, I assert that as part of our agreement, I will help them free themselves, and guide and encourage them in ways that have proven helpful with others. I play down my role. Instead of transferring their buried and painful emotions to me, it is *far more effective* if they connect these emotions in fantasy with the significant people with whom they have developed emotional conflicts!

This change of emphasis radically increases the speed and effectiveness with which a person grows. Now I, as the therapist, become an ally of the healthy Self of the patient, encouraging patients to free themselves from their own inner enemies. We work to re-create that core of wholeness with which the patient was born and de-emphasize the patient's self-image as "sick" or "neurotic." The Self on the Personality Chart becomes a star to steer by. Disturbed people lack self-esteem, a central part of the problem. When regarded by the therapist as fundamentally whole with the capacity to grow, patients increase their ability to challenge their own self-defeating attitudes.

This may seem abstract and theoretical to you. Let me reassure you, however, that as we soon move on to suggesting actual techniques for your own emotional self-liberation, things will become very real indeed. You will actually be able to experience the use of sounds and movements to free your tensions and blocked emotions, and you will experience your "rage to live" as a positive force you have never tapped before.

Although the neurotic processes described on the Personality Chart are not a part of the real Self, they must be challenged and overcome or they will keep the real Self buried and cripple the potential for health, vitality, and happiness. To liberate energy, I encourage the patient to express whatever sounds and movements have been bound up in inner tension. I call this process "the language of emotion." This process fulfills Freud's prophecies and extends Reich's work. Syntonic therapy has accelerated the therapeutic process that so often gets bogged down in talking till doomsday, and it has enabled many people who have been abandoned as inaccessible by conventional psychoanalysts and psychiatrists to free themselves.

Helping patients challenge and overcome their defenses and release their fear, sadness, and anger enables them to focus on their inner problems rather than transfer them to the therapist. The real enemies are within: the old tensions and blocked emotions; the images and unhealed experiences that limit one's freedom in the present moment. As patients express the anger and rage they feel in the language of emotion, they progressively learn to direct these negative emotions against the parts of themselves that are self-defeating and gradually slough off the debris that has buried the real Self. The energy of anger has the power to dissolve fear and hopelessness. Those people whose anger and rage are buried are passive individuals, depressed and "down in the mouth." Until they emotionally "get it off their chest," they never come alive.

The important thing to remember is that *it is all right to feel whatever you feel.* It is all right to express these feelings, without hurting yourself or others. The beginning of growth is indicated when a patient begins to express fearful and helpless sounds, or sad sounds with sobbing (sometimes with words that are meaningful and integrated with feeling). This starts the syntonic process of unifying ("syn") the person and affords release, strengthening of the personality, and increased aliveness and self-esteem.

Gradually, over a period of weeks and months, sounds of annoyance and angry feelings and movements will appear as energy is thawed out from the state of being "scared stiff" or "petrified with fear." Expressing this by pounding or stamping cushions can also be integrating and strengthening.

For example, a patient named Bill came to me for Syntonic therapy after having had five analysts and as many types of therapy over a period of twenty years. His condition was depressed and hopeless. He was caught in rounds of compulsive homosexuality, drinking, smoking, pill taking, and overeating. Though he talked endlessly about his deep terror of dying, of being abandoned and rejected (he had had a sickly, helpless childhood), Bill never was able to release his acute fears. I helped him to understand that he was clinging to his self-pity, spite, and suffering.[3]

Using the language of emotion to extricate himself, Bill gradually grew from a moaning, helpless baby to a furious child. I helped him to turn his rage from himself to the parts of himself which he hated, such as his own masochistic tendencies, which were a repetition of his father's cruelty toward him as a child. Bill slowly destroyed the cruel "father" image within himself. Similarly, his self-pampering (derived from his mother) dissolved as he destroyed the negative facet of the inner "mother" image. He ended his addictions, became able to enjoy being alone, learned to be positively assertive, and for the first time established a normal and enjoyable sexual relationship with a woman he cared for. His entire posture and manner changed as he employed his rage as a *positive force* to conquer his tensions and fears. At last he found the self-respect that is a natural part of one's real Self.

Bill had feared his rage and had masochistically directed it to himself, with endless self-criticism. He had also turned his rage on his previous doctors, and through covert spite had thwarted their attempts to help him. Once he began to accept his rage as *his own power* and learned to experience this rage fully and direct it productively, he had the key to his own liberation. Happily, as he grew, he became more

---

[3] R. Kronemeyer, *Overcoming Homosexuality*, Macmillan Pub. Co., N.Y., Collier Macmillan Pub., London, 1980.

understanding, forgiving, and loving toward his parents!

The mental aspect of Syntonic therapy—the use of thoughts and images—will be explored in the following section.

A Hard Look at Your Body's Emotions

Before you start to practice your exercises for emotional liberation, spend a few moments before a long mirror—if possible, in the nude.

First, look at your face. Can you look into your eyes directly, or do you look away? Do your eyes and facial expression tend to be frightened or troubled or sad? Does your forehead tend to be wrinkled in worry? Do your mouth and jaw have a set attitude, a resigned or angry look? Your face will provide clues about emotions which may be known to you only superficially. Such emotions need no longer be buried inside to disturb your well-being; they can be released by means of the exercises suggested in the section on mobilizing your energy starting on page 140.

Notice how you hold your head. Is it held forward? Is it held up in the air? Does your head tend to have a downcast hang-dog look? How does each of these attitudes make you feel? Now balance your head upright. Holding your head forward characterizes a fearful attitude. Holding it in a haughty manner is being "above it all" or denying your fear. Thus, we talk of stiff-necked pride. Being centered only in your head, rather than in the real center of gravity below the navel, *does* make you physically and emotionally unbalanced. Such people go from flying high in grandiosity to feeling low and worthless.

Notice how your pelvis is set. Are your buttocks held back in a tight and controlled position? Are they collapsed forward? Or are they balanced in a comfortable position in between? The placement of your pelvis can indicate emotional conflicts about sexuality.

Observe the attitude of your shoulders. Do they hang down hopelessly? Are they hunched up as if fearful and protective? Perhaps they are stiff, held with a "chip on the shoulder," carrying anger. Are your shoulders balanced a relaxed in a natural and pleasurable position?

Now look at your posture. Do you lock your knees stiffly, or do you stand in a relaxed manner with a looseness about the knees? Do you slouch on one side or the other? As you release tension by exhaling completely and bring energy down through your body by stamping, you will begin to feel more securely grounded, with a solid foundation for your being. You will be able to "take a stand" and to "put your foot down" with yourself and others. *The root of emotional and mental health is in your pelvis, legs, and feet.* After you practice the emotional release exercises for several weeks (see page 142), look at yourself again in a long mirror. You will see changes taking place in your posture and in your emotional attitudes, and you will witness the growth of your dignity, self-respect, and aliveness.

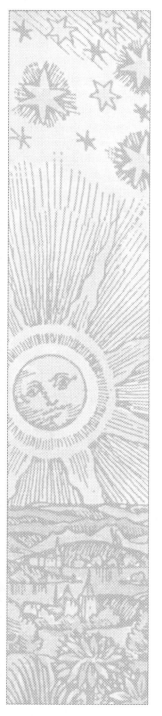

EIGHT

Emotional Techniques for Freeing Yourself

Human emotions can be powerful forces for good or ill in our daily lives. Plato compared a human being to a horse-drawn chariot and a driver. The driver represents human thinking and the power of reason; the swift steed represents the motivating strength of human emotions. When our horse-power or emotions are sluggish, we feel depressed; when they are skittish, we feel anxious; when they kick and bite, we feel hostile; when they are flighty, we become elated—only to fall back with fatigue into another depressed state. But when our feelings are flowing and in syntony with the driver—our reason—we can move constructively toward our goals and enjoy the time given to us. A wise Indian medicine man once said to me, "Death is at our shoulder and can tap us at any moment—so there is no time for negative thoughts or moods." The best antidote to death is to live fully. Then, when death comes one can say, "So be it—nothing lasts forever, and I have enjoyed the gift of life and the adventure of living and growing."

Because we live in a tense and disturbed world, it is easy to slip into negative emotional states, to become chronically anxious, sad, and angry. We can be consumed by these emotions without having an outlet for them and then be driven into other destructive behaviors and habits, which lead to a vicious circle of guilt, physical illness, self-hatred, fatigue, and depression.

The purpose of this chapter is to start you on the path away from negativity and toward the benevolent circle, so that gradually you can understand some of the roots of these negative emotions in your life and learn to release them in the present without harm. Sometimes we can feel so upset and confused that it is wise to seek a trained therapist for assistance. When you need help, it is healthy to seek it. By all means, find a wholistic therapist who deals with all aspects of health. However, when we are disturbed, we tend to run away from the very help we need because of fear and distrust. Often we blame others for the suffering we are either creating or allowing others to put on us.

As you can see in the Personality Chart, often in our earliest years we lose the syntony and well-being with which we are born. This happens because as infants and children, the tremendous needs we have for love, security, and respect for our natural emotions are rarely satisfied in our society. Gradually, we slip into the unholy trinity of fear, sadness, and anger as we lose our undisturbed state of wholeness and inner freedom.

We all have experienced this painful state. We must learn to help ourselves avoid it or, when confronted by it, to regain a loving energy flow as quickly as possible. When we feel anxious without real cause or allow ourselves to sink into hopelessness, we also create anger or hatred within. When one of these negative emotions appears, others may be hidden in the shadows. It is not surprising that "the devil" is often depicted as having a hunched body, fearful and hateful emotional attitudes, a cunning and devious mind, and a spirit that is cut off from the creative power of love—the quintessence of this negative state!

Sounds for Emotional Release

How can we use our emotional power to regain a freer and happier state of being? A child can show us the way. As children, we used what I call the language of emotions before we learned words. We used sounds and movements to release our emotional tensions. We screamed or cried out our fear; we cried and sobbed with sadness; we kicked, yelled, and flailed our arms with anger. Often these natural reactions were punished rather than regarded as a call for help and reassurance. Thus, we were driven to the defenses described in the Personality Chart. When these defenses against our negative feelings subsequently prove inadequate, we develop the various physical, emotional, mental, and spiritual symptoms that accompany our lack of harmony and syntony.

Mobilize Your Energy by Letting
Your Anger Out

Sounds are one tool by which you can release emotional tension and breathe more deeply. For privacy when trying this exercise, you may want to close the door to your bedroom, play a radio, and muffle any spontaneous sounds you might express by means of a rolled-up towel or pillow. (If you have privacy, let the sounds come as they will.) Sounds of fear can release fearful tensions. Sounds of sadness or crying can free your despair. Sounds of anger can liberate tension that you might otherwise take out on yourself or loved ones. Your strongest outgoing emotion, next to love, is anger. Syntonic therapy utilizes anger to overcome fear and hopelessness in *the transition to love*.

If images of people from the past or present come into your awareness, direct your emotions at these images. Remember that in your relationship with your parents, you had both loving *and* negative feelings at different times. Unfortunately, you were cautioned against feeling anger toward them while being coaxed to feel only love for them. But at times parents can be frightening, mean, impatient, and disappointing—and they may deserve your anger. Parents are not perfect! Accept that you contain *all* these feelings toward your parents *within you*. This truth can begin to set you free emotionally.

As you release sounds, and the tensions and emotions that accompany them, you will find that your tension, sadness, and anger are lessened. Your breath will flow freely and your body will be more relaxed. Never blame yourself for any emotions you may feel, for they are the result of hurts you suffered at various times in your life. Often after releasing negative feelings and destroying the negative images connected with people close to you, you will be able to feel more understanding, compassionate, and loving toward them. Bottled-up negative emotions always block our deeper positive emotions!

Having released all this tension, make pleasurable sounds—sighs of relief, for example. Soft sounds come when you are connected with the center of your being through deeper breathing and inner awareness.

Using Sounds to Release Tension and Blocked Emotions

- Choose a room where you can turn on music for soundproofing and not be concerned about being heard.
- Stretch out on a bed with a pillow at hand.
- Make sounds into the pillow, and feel what emotion (fear, anger, sadness, joy, etc.) is coming forth.
- Breathe deeply and go with the feeling until you feel a sense of relief.
- If you feel stuck in fear or sadness, mobilize anger to move through that painful and helpless state by yelling in the pillow: "I hate feeling afraid!"; "I hate feeling weak! [or hopeless, sad, etc.]" Then pound the pillow with positive anger.
- Yell strongly positive affirmations: "I can be free!" "I will feel good!" "I am worthwhile!" etc. Stamp as you yell.
- If you feel you cannot handle these emotions, seek a therapist who is not afraid to work with emotions as well as thoughts.

Movements for Emotional Release

Body movements help release negative emotions, as sounds do. Infants and young children instinctively know this. Allow warm and pleasant feelings to move your body in pleasurable ways. Stretch out toward the world with your lips, arms, and hands. If you still retain anxiety, sadness, or anger, lie on your back, hold the sides of the bed, bring one knee up toward your chest, and kick your leg out parallel to the bed as you exhale sharply. This process can help liberate fear, tension, sadness, and anger. If negative images come to mind, kick out against these images. You have created these images: They are nourished by your energy, and you have the right to free yourself of them. Though we do not have the right to attack others, we do have the right to destroy inner negative images that accompany a disturbed emotional state. Remember the expression "to kick the habit." To have the will to become free, you must mobilize energy to strengthen your willpower—to kick out neurotic habits ingrained as patterns of unreasonable fear, hopelessness, and anger.

If you feel stuck at the present time, remember that in every living organism there is a will to live which, when blocked, becomes a "rage to live." The worst mistake you can make is to turn that rage against yourself; another serious mistake is to turn that rage against other people. Rage can be a powerful instrument. Turn that rage against your inner enemies (i.e., those physical tensions you allow to bind you; the fear or hopelessness or self-pity that you allow to cripple your freedom; the negative parental images and thoughts that you allow to deplete your energy).

To forgive means "to go past." In forgiving, you will also go past your own fearful and hostile state. Only the strong can genuinely forgive. As long as we remain crippled, vengeful, and weak, forgiveness is not possible. Forgiveness comes with freedom — an attribute of the Life Force. This is a challenging realization. The more powerful your negative feelings, the more power you have accessible with which to free yourself from your inner enemies!

To alleviate tension in your neck, shoulders, and back, kneel on your bed with a pillow in front of you. Reaching back as far as you can with two fists, pound the pillow with a sharp exhalation. Accompany this with a sound like a karate master breaking a board. If you become aware of any images connected with fear or hostility, make those images your imaginary target. Otherwise, focus your rage to live on your tension. As you hit, say "I'm tired of being afraid," "I'm tired of being negative," or whatever else you are tired of keeping locked in yourself.

Affirmative Stamping

"Putting your foot down" about aspects of yourself that you wish to stamp out can also help you free energy for growth. Place several foam cushions on the floor, and stamp strongly as you exhale. Say the things you are tired of in yourself as you stamp: "I hate anxiety, procrastination, pettiness, spite, etc." Then assert each attitude you wish to strengthen as you *stamp in a positive and assertive way.* For example: "I am worthwhile"; "I will assert myself"; "I can open my heart and love"; "I am one with God" . . . etc.

The Magic of Positive Imagery

Having released negative emotions it is important to *rechannel* your energy in a healthy way to create positive emotions. This is the second part of Syntonic therapy: the use of *positive imagery*. Remember: one must pull the weeds *and* cultivate one's garden.

Sitting relaxed and upright, picture yourself in a happy and lively mood. See yourself as warm and positive, and as you breathe easily and deeply into the center of your being, feel gently loving feelings flowing from this center. Picture these warm vibrations flowing out toward the invisible infinite Life Force around you, the very source of your life and existence. Next picture and feel these warm energy currents flowing from the Source to every cell of your body, in a caring and loving way. Enjoy the feeling of respecting and loving yourself. Picture the Life Force flowing from your center out through every part of your body toward every person on the planet. If there are people you cannot yet accept and love, feel compassion toward them and picture them as you would like them to be. In this way, each time you do this exercise you can fulfill the two conditions that will assure you a rich and abundant life free of fear and hatred: eliminating the negative and cultivating the positive. Is there any better, freer or happier state of being?

Humans have a two-sided nervous system; one side whose function is to run or fight in fear or hate like a coiled up hissing cat; the other to experience joy and relaxation like a cat purring with pleasure. The Bible teaches: (1st John 4:18) "Love casts out fear," a truth validated 2000 years later by the discovery of this autonomic nervous system! After you release your negative attitudes this healthy state can be cultivated through the use of positive imagery. The core of physical, emotional, mental and spiritual health is the loving state, in which energy flows toward the Cosmic Power, toward yourself and others. We have been given the gift of life. We have also been given the privilege of freedom. Whether we use or misuse our precious share of the Life Energy in happiness or misery is our own responsibility and choice.

The practice of these exercises will propel you toward emotional growth and inner security. You will gradually be able to handle difficult life situations with positive assertion rather than with fear and submission or rage and desperation. If your tendency has been to cling to destructive jobs or relationships, you will begin to have the courage to change or abandon sterile situations. If you have reacted to difficulties with nastiness or hostility, you will learn to assert yourself in a positive way. This will add to your self-respect and the respect of others. Remember: Growth takes patience, vigilance, and effort.

Take a moment now to use positive imagery to picture yourself handling some difficult situation or relationship as you remain in a loving state of being. The more strongly you feel this way, the more clearly you can picture yourself acting assertively and positively, the more easily you will handle your problem in actuality. If, having behaved reasonably and assertively, you do lose the job or relationship, you will have lost little of real value and at the same time will have gained something priceless—greater self-respect. Before you deal with any difficult life situation, be sure that you are focused in your center of gravity, just below your navel, the locus of your real Self. In this state, you will be strong and reasonable and flexible. When you lose this settled-down state by acting out the role of a frightened child or an uptight negative patent, you become either weak and impotent or rigid and explosive. Practice positive imagery so that, whether among your family or with other people, you will enjoy being a balanced human being, with your feet on the ground.

You deserve your fullest development. Use positive imagery to picture yourself being free of those habits or parts of yourself that you wish to outgrow. In this way, you will avoid the habit of being negatively self-critical; and you will develop the mature ability to help yourself grow — in the way a stable and loving parent helps a child: in this case your "inner child."

We all carry over "baggage from our past" — habits and attitudes which are inappropriate in the present. Changing is not easy, and when patients complain about how difficult it is, I say there is one thing much more difficult: staying immature and miserable.

Since your inner child did not get as much love and understanding as needed — for a plethora of reasons — now *you* can be a loving parent to your inner child.

- Take a pillow and hug it to your heart, as you would a child who needed love and understanding; give a name to your inner child.
- In doing so, you will be opening your heart to loving feelings which will free you from fear and negativity.
- Be loving but firm to your inner child (the two requisites of good parenting) and explain out loud that from now on you (your adult self) are taking over in a positive way.
- Review the nine defenses on the Personality Chart and the attitudes that are counterproductive and undesirable.
- Choose the ones that relate to you, and explain to your inner child that together you are going to work on eliminating them.
- For example, if you tend to be passive and give up easily, tell your inner child that you are going to

change this and stick to things and give up immediate satisfaction for longer-range gratification.

- If you tend to be spiteful and procrastinate in a self-damaging way, be assertive with your inner child and make it clear that you are going to oppose this habit strongly and get positive satisfaction for avoiding stress, guilt, and embarrassment and doing things on time.

- By giving love, you can relieve whatever fear, sadness, anger, guilt, or shame your inner child and you may be suffering from.

These two principles—eliminating the negative and rechanneling energy into the positive—will enable you to change and overcome any pattern of thought, feeling, or behavior you wish. First release the tension, fear, and negative thinking that drive you to indulge in self-destructive habits. Each time you "pull the weeds," spend several minutes cultivating your garden. As you picture yourself feeling and behaving in a free and natural way, you will be strengthening the benevolent circle while moving toward health, happiness, and a rich and meaningful life.

What Is This Thing Called Love?

Love is a word that is often used and often abused. Bogus love is always egoistic and concerned with getting rather than giving. It can be a mask for possessiveness or clinging out of fear, or for dominating another person for one's own sexual, emotional, or distorted psychological needs!

The art of loving begins with being a loving person—loving life as a whole and oneself as part of it. Genuine love is expansive and never exclusive, for it is an attitude, a

personal orientation toward the Life Force that has respect
for creation itself. If you lack this spiritual attitude and
claim to love a particular person, your love is not mature but
is selfish, desperate, and exploitative. For respect is always
the basic ingredient of authentic love. Those who have not
found their Self (see the Personality Chart) can only use
others to "make me happy," which never works. Just as
vitality is the characteristic of physical health, love is the
fulfillment of emotional maturity. Love is quite rare at this
stage of human development. But it is priceless, and it is
worthy of cultivation by overcoming the tensions, fears, and
hatred that imprison it.

Carl is an example of a man who thought he "loved"
Mary, and to prove his love he insisted that she was so
important in his life that he "could not live without her."

But not being able to live without another person is a
state of dependency characteristic of infancy and childhood! Though a successful stockbroker, Carl was still a
child emotionally. Coddled and overprotected by his
mother, and lacking a father capable of giving him caring
and positive discipline, he had never grown up.

In genuine adulthood, it is *appropriate* to be dependent on
the Higher Power that created us and sustains us at every
moment. That is what humility is all about. But to make
another finite being God is totally unrealistic. Mary could
not accept the possessive and jealous demands that Carl
placed on her, and she sought to escape from this suffocat-
ing situation. Feeling rejected after having given Mary
"everything," Carl threatened to kill himself. This made
him realize finally that he had deep problem to deal with if
he were ever to have a secure and happy relationship. It
gradually dawned on him that until one is happy with oneself and in harmony with the Higher Power, one is not

ready to relate to anyone else in a positive way. No wonder so few marriages at this stage of human development are truly fulfilling.

In *The Art of Loving*, written by Dr. Erich Fromm in 1954, Fromm stresses the importance of respect as the crucial ingredient of love. Respect means "to see a person as he is, to be aware of his unique individuality, and to be concerned that "the other person should grow and unfold as he is," and "not for the purpose of serving me."

Carl struggled to outgrow his fears and to achieve independence. He used syntonic release techniques every day, changed his diet and lifestyle, worked with the Syntonic cassette tape every day and practiced aikido meditation frequently. This self-therapy greatly speeded up his progress toward regaining his authentic Self (see Personality Chart). As he slowly grew in inner security and self-respect, he finally became ready for a mature relationship based on love and respect rather than fear and exploitation.

Body language is a clear expression of the contrast between the fear/hate orientation of survival, (the fight or flight reaction) and the positive outgoing love orientation. In the former, when we are threatened, we tense up ready to run or attack with explosive force. In loving, however, we open our hearts and our bodies as we reach out to embrace a parent, a child, a friend or God.

In the Western tradition, one kind of love is *eros*. This includes the sexual energy or libido and is the drive to procreate. When this involves the heart, we call it making love, which involves a caring for the loved one. Without that caring only lust remains, and instead of the re-creative power of true love making, the *mysterium tremendum*, there is a tension release at best and a sense of emptiness and meaningless at worst; rutting leaves the soul unsatisfied.

A second form of love is *philia*, or friendship, brotherly love. The third form of love is *agape*, in the Greek tradition, (*caritas* as the Romans called it). In both of these there is a caring, and a heartfelt respect for the other but without a libidinal element. In genuine love, there is a flow outward as an invisible stream of energy from the spiritual reservoir of one's deepest Self. In sharp contrast, desire is a taking in by the needy ego. Thus we say, to honor this power that comprises our connection with the Life Force Itself, "God is Love."

By chance I came upon a book in my library by the Spanish philosopher Ortega y Gasset.[1] The title *On Love* caught my eye. Discovering a commonality of thought and spirit with great minds is a cardinal joy of the intellectual life. I tingled as I read his words

"Love is a flow, a stream of spiritual matter, a fluid that flows continually like a fountain. . . . Love is not an explosion, but a continued emanation, a psychic radiation which proceeds from the lover to the beloved." Here the beloved can be one's child, one's friend, one's spouse, one's parent, or one's Creator. When it includes libidinal energy, the beloved becomes one's lover. But sexuality without the spiritual dimension, merely on an animal level, is like comparing a hut to a castle.

Ortega goes on to delineate the difference between love and hate mirroring my own point of view. "Since they are centrifugal, both love and hate move in the same direction, the person involved going toward the object; nevertheless, in spite of sharing the same direction, their reasoning and

---

[1] Ortega y Gasset, J., *On Love* (trans. by Toby Talbot), Meridian Books. Cleveland and N.Y., 1957 (From the original text, Estudios sobre el amor).

intention are different. In hate, the reason being negative one goes toward the object but against it. In love, one also goes toward the object but on its behalf."

Across time and space I send a flowing stream from my heart of *philia* and *agape* toward Ortega y Gasset, my brother whom I have never met, and my fellow spirit with whom I shall always be at onement.

Fifteen Steps to Strengthening Your Emotional Health in Self-Therapy

Part 1: Pulling the Weeds the Syntonic Way

1. Choose a time when you have a room to yourself with no outside interference. Kneel in front of cushions on the bed or floor. Bring your awareness to your inner being, and determine your emotional state. If you feel sad, discouraged, or lonely and cut off from life, take a rolled-up towel and release into it the sounds of hurt or pain that you are feeling, releasing this inner tension as strongly as possible. If you can cry deeply, so much the better. This may lead to your inner child telling one or both of your inner parents how you feel about the way they treated you. (Even if they have passed on, the painful, negative feelings you have toward them must be worked through.) Or your tears may help you see the negative parts of your immature or lower self (fear, spite, pettiness, greed, false pride, laziness, anger, egotism, etc.). Ask your deeper Self to help you overcome these self-destructive attitudes.

2. If you are more in touch with frustrations, tension,

and rage, breathe deeply and go with these feelings by letting out expressive sounds (and words, if they come spontaneously). You can also make two fists, reach back as far as you can, and then bring your fists forward and strike the pillows in front of you as you sharply exhale. Or, as you lie on your back, bring one knee in toward your chest and drive it out as strongly as you can with each exhalation. Where there is anxiety (chronic tension and fear), there is always sadness, because it is sad to be cut off from life. And there is always rage (although it is often unconscious and buried under depression), because to be alienated from love (the joyful flow of the Life Force) is painful on all levels of our being—physical, emotional, mental, and spiritual. Of course, it is easier in the short run to fall back on your addiction when you are experiencing anxiety and disease (alcohol, caffeine, sugar, nicotine, food, compulsive sexuality, drugs, etc.). The way out of the vicious circle is to convince yourself that for a *pittance* of relief you are choosing a life that is *95 percent pain.*

3. When you feel frightened or sad, hold a pillow to your heart and, as you hug your inner child, express in tender words and carresses the love that you wish you had received. With this love and support, your inner child will at last be able to outgrow its fear, hurt, and sadness.

4. To strengthen the energy flow from your pelvis downward, leading toward more sexual maturity and independence, lie down and kick out with the same thoughts and feelings as when you pounded previously.

5. Place the cushions on the floor, and as you stamp on them, connect your thoughts and words with the thoughts and attitudes that you dislike in yourself or in others. This, too, helps restore the syntony, or wholeness, that is your birthright and the very essence of self-esteem, strength, and happiness—the unity of mind, body, emotions, and spirit: your soul.

6. You will have to repeat the cathartic exercises a number of times, but each repetition will make you stronger and more unified. As you release the frozen energy of fear, anger, and sadness, you will gradually evolve toward your whole Self and be able to express your anger cleanly when appropriate in a strong, assertive fashion, and then *resume* your healthy inner state of joy and love. In chronic fear and rage, we are torn with conflict over whether to fight, flee, or submit. Only in a relaxed and loving state can we enjoy inner freedom and peace.

7. Remember, your rage may connect with negative aspects of your parents or others that you have good reason to hate. You have the right to express whatever you want to in dealing with hateful aspects of the people who hurt you, *even if those people meant well.* You need not trap yourself in self-punishing, guilty thoughts and feelings. You can also love the positive aspects of those same people. Knowing and accepting this will free you to use the power of your rage as a positive force to free yourself gradually from anxiety, sadness, negativity, guilt, and lack of self-esteem. Only as hate is released and understood can forgiveness and love flow.

Most of these strong feelings relate not to your parents in the present day, but to the parents you perceived in infancy and childhood, when your misconceptions and negative reactions (the best you could muster at the time) added to the inter-personal problems. Therefore, much of this rage should be taken out on *the images* of your parents which you carry in your mind, and not on your parents directly. Of course, as you grow stronger, self-assertive feelings are appropriate toward any-one—parents included.

8. It is also important to focus your rage on attitudes and behavior patterns that you know are childish (the ones suggested in the first paragraph of this section). Whether you lie down and kick, or stand up and stamp, or kneel and pound, try to direct the flow of strong emotional energy to challenge these negative patterns. Let the feeling be expressed in words: "I'm tired of . . ." "I hate . . ." "I'm through with . . ." However, *never* direct hate toward your-self. You are a creation of God. Direct it only toward the aspects of yourself that disturb your well-being.

9. You may want to ask the help of a good friend who understands the need to release negative emotions in order to free the basic positive energy. If the path toward wholeness seems too steep, lonely, or frightening to travel by yourself, look for someone to stand by you. Or find a therapist who will help you use the power of your emotions instead of cut-ting you off from them by analysis and suppres-sion. Keep in mind that the Higher Power is *always there* to help you discover the inner truth, and "the

truth will set you free." But remember that you cannot coast to freedom; effort and perseverance are necessary.

Part 2: Cultivating the Garden the Syntonic Way

10. After a session with yourself, finish as we do in Syntonic therapy sessions, by strengthening your true and healthy Self. You can practice centering, as described in Chapter 4, and expressing the positive affirmations that come from your heart at the moment. Finish the session by visualizing your new and positive Self relating to your own being, the world, people around you, and God in a loving and assertive way.

11. Remember, if you are unhappy, *only you* are keeping yourself in that state or allowing another person to do so. Only you are blocking the flow of the Life Force, which is an infinite source of freedom, pleasure, and love. "Where the Spirit of the Lord is, there is freedom." (II Corinthians, 3:17) So if you give up your arrogance and challenge your laziness, you will find that you have really lost nothing and have gained everything. But the choice is yours. We reap what we sow.

12. If you wish to create your own cassette for emotional well-being, you can recite the following, as I did when I made my own cassette or add to it.

To concretize my birthright, emotional health, and well-being, I affirm that
  I am One with the Creative Power of the Universe. I experience that Oneness with every breath.
Every breath is a gift of Life Energy from the Infinite.

I love the Holy Spirit that flows through me. It opens my
  heart with joy and happiness.
I am awake to the miracle of creation.
My feeling of love is more precious than all the wealth in
  the world.
The more I help others, the better I feel.
In oneness, I am free from separation and loneliness.
As my love strengthens, my fear diminishes.
My heart feels light as I forgive those who have hurt me.
My body, emotions, mind, and spirit are in harmony.
I am filled with kindness, pleasure, and love.
I am free of distorted thoughts and addictions.
Every day I grow in freedom and joy.
The more I love life and others, the more I love myself.

13. Remember, it is necessary to pull the weeds; to face
    and work through the negative attitudes that we
    carry from the past, which are often hidden from
    others and from ourselves as well. But if you use
    these methods, you will succeed, because your true
    Self wants to come forth, and you will suffer in
    many ways until it does.

    Gradually, you will notice that the release of strong
    feeling becomes less violent as tensions lessen, and
    your level of well-being will increase. You will
    spend more time in Self-cultivation as you become
    emotionally more free and happy.

14. Have no doubt! The more you *concretize* your
    healthy Self emotionally, with affirmations from
    your heart, and the more you *visualize* yourself
    being that kind of person, the more you will *actu-
    alize* emotional health in your daily life.

15. For those who find it difficult to use these active
    techniques to release and dissolve suppressed and

repressed anger and hostility, "hate letters" can be very effective. These letters will not, of course, be sent; they can even be written to a deceased parent toward whom you harbor mixed emotions that are destructively *transferred* to unfortunate people you interact with *in the present*. Without holding back, express fully the hate you carry toward parents or other significant people in your life. Read over these letters for three days, out loud if you wish, and then burn them, page by page. Visualize your hatred going up in smoke; and then in a dialogue with each person, ask forgiveness for *your part* in the negative interaction. Finally, visualize yourself with these people in a centered and secure state of being, able to be assertive and understanding; no longer trapped in fear, guilt, and hostility.

The Human Mind

The mind is like a monkey
on a tree endlessly chattering and
jumping about.

—HINDU SAYING

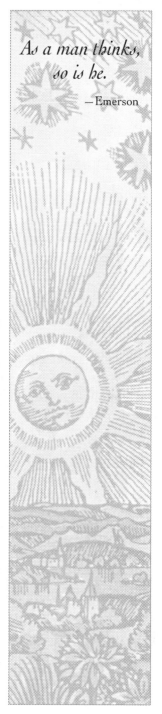

*As a man thinks,
so is he.*

—Emerson

NINE

Understanding the Disturbed Mind

I believe that the Greek philosophers were correct in asserting that "a sound mind in a sound body" are inseparable. Conversely, the tense and disturbed body of the neurotic individual is always accompanied by a disturbed mind. We have seen that the tense body harbors fear, anger, and sadness, which stem from a lack of adequate love during infancy and which evolve into reactions of hurt and protest during childhood that rejecting parents subsequently punish rather than understand.

Wholistic reeducation deals with the body and emotions as well as the mind. Dr. Janov who created the famous phrase "the primal scream" describes just one of many aspects of mental disturbance: "Tension operates in the mind as incoherence, confusion, and lack of memory, and in the body as tight musculature and distortions of the visceral process."

The Anxious Mind

The mind mediates between the inner being and the outer world. Neurotic minds (like neurotic people) are compulsively busy and restless—driven by underlying anxiety, they are incapable of a peaceful moment. The *anxious* mind perceives reality as fearful and dangerous. Since neurotic people are afraid of adult goals, their thinking is obsessively concerned with safety. Still a dependent "child," they invent ways to please others so they will be considered a good child to mother and father figures. Caught in negative judgments of their past that have long been programmed within them, they worry endlessly. What if this happens, and what if that happens?

But healthy people see good possibilities and are willing to risk disappointment as part of the experience of living. Since they value themselves, their self-worth is not at stake. The neurotic mind of anxious individuals always expects the worst to happen, and until this basic fear is resolved, no amount of positive experience will convince them that their thinking is one-sided. Therapies and religious teachings that stress positive thinking may be helpful, but for neurotic individuals they have limited value—it is like spraying the leaves of a plant without nourishing the roots. Both the thought processes as well as the whole *person* need to be helped toward integration and syntony.

The Hostile Mind

The Roman philosopher Epictetus is reputed to have said, "Men are not disturbed by events, but by their attitude toward them." Whereas the person with an anxious mental attitude is overly concerned with his or her own safety ("better safe than sorry") the overly aggressive person is ruled by a sadistic mental attitude obsessed with power and tends to act in a ruthless and predatory manner. Preoccupied with hostile thoughts and fed by inner tension and rage (transferred from hated parents to members of society), this hostile inner child who has adult intelligence often becomes a criminal. Grandiose fantasies that derive from inner feelings of worthlessness are acted out, and thus a criminal psychopath such as Hitler can rise to power.

When socialization (upbringing and education) produces a sufficient number of hostile and passive followers (both created in the autocratic family), the psychopath's success is ensured.[1]

Dr. Kurt Lewin's studies of autocratic and democratic group dynamics reveal this process. The boys he studied were more hostile and less self-directing under bossy leaders than they were with democratic leaders. How long could a fanatic such as Hitler flourish in a healthy and loving society?

The drive to conquer expresses itself in the manipulation and exploitation of others and is driven by fear, hostility, and the absence of compassion and self-esteem. The obsessive need for prestige and endless material possessions becomes such a person's paramount concern. One's meaning in life becomes the "bitch goddess success," and this

---

[1] Kurt Lewin, *Group Dynamics* (3rd edition), Harper and Row, N.Y., 1968, p. 318.

mania becomes all-consuming. Countless examples of such
driven minds exist in every walk of life, from the arts and
sciences to industry and politics. Never having had genuine
love and acceptance, such unbalanced people are never satisfied no matter what the extent of their conquests.
Sexually, such compulsion is characteristic of nymphoman-
ics and satyromaniacs.

The Withdrawn Mind

Individuals who withdraw tend to flee from the life struggle. As part of the animal kingdom, humans share the fundamental survival reactions of submission, fight, or flight.
Neurosis is a conditioning toward one main tendency,
which becomes "characteristic" or, as Wilhelm Reich
defined in *Character Analysis*, "the way of reacting that has
become structure."[2] Every basically fearful person has all
these conflicting tendencies, though one trait becomes most
apparent. The mind of the withdrawn person, overwhelmed
with pessimism, seeks victory in defeat. The mind becomes
more or less detached from the threatening outer world and
from painful feelings of fear, sadness, and rage. Fantasy
vividly becomes the artificial reality of this type, in which
the grandiose and heroic self can conquer and achieve,
escape from the pain of the "bad child," and compensate for
the lost inner peace and sense of self-worth of the essential
Self. Constant suppression of hurt and anger, which were
punished in childhood, develops into that process which
Reich named armoring[3] (i.e., the locking off and denial of

---

[2] Wilhelm Reich, *Character Analysis*, Orgone Institute Press, N.Y., 1949, p. 218.
[3] Wilhelm Reich, op. cit. p. 70.

these emotions and the painful memories which accompany them). Freud understood that constant suppression became repression, and forbidden thoughts and feelings fell into the unconscious mind:

> Above all [is] the great thinker Schopenhauer, whose unconscious "will" is equivalent to the instincts in the mind as seen by psychoanalysis. It was this same thinker, moreover, who in words of unforgettable impressiveness admonished mankind of the importance of their sexual craving, still so depricated.[4]

The healthy, secure individual is in touch with inner positive feelings and with outer reality. Imagination and fantasy are used creatively to conceive satisfying and realistic goals. In the detached person, inner feelings are too painful and guilt provoking; because the real world is too frightening, imagination creates a "new world" in which fulfillment can be achieved (it is hoped) magically, with neither risk nor effort. Such fantasies charge the mind with a temporary elation, which is soon followed by depression as the energy is withdrawn and the person once again feels stuck and helpless. Lacking a sense of wholeness, assertion, and centeredness, the detached person tends to live in his or her troubled and overburdened head (the universal gesture for mental illness, logically, is the forefinger pointing toward the temple and turning in circles, mimicking the cerebral whirlpool of the restless mind). Thus, the term *head shrinker* refers to one who cures mental unrest and helps the patient restore peace of mind.

---

[4] Wilhelm Reich, op. cit. p. 380.[fo]

Test Your Mental Health

Take this quiz to determine the state of your own mental health. Put a check mark beside the statements that apply to you.

I tend to:

- withdraw from new situations _____
- daydream about things I want _____
- envy people who seem happy _____
- enjoy secret grandiose fantasies _____
- think negatively about myself _____
- be constantly worried _____
- be bothered by compulsive thoughts _____
- get obsessed about certain people _____
- ask God to do things for me _____
- be disturbed by sadistic thoughts _____
- think negatively about others _____
- tell myself other people *must* like me _____
- be disturbed by masochistic thoughts _____
- overreact to disappointments _____
- demand perfection of myself _____
- be selfish and self-centered _____
- get trapped in procrastination _____
- either be too passive or too aggressive _____
- lie even when I do not want to _____
- hurt myself with addictions I can't conquer _____

For every characteristic that applies to you, give yourself one point. The lower the score, the better. Under five is a good score; five to ten is fair; ten to fifteen indicates a need for self-help or outside counseling; and higher than fifteen indicates a serious need for therapy.

The Neurotic Thought Process

In neurosis of all kinds and degrees, the mind loses its capacity to be aware of inner and outer reality, and instead twists or denies reality to avoid hurt and danger. There are methods to all madness. Clinging and dependent people rationalize, "Look how loyal I am; I've given you the best years of my life," and they try to blame someone for using them while hiding the fact that they were also using the other person for support. Overaggressive types justify their behavior with, "It's a dog-eat-dog world, and I'd rather be top dog than under dog," hiding the fact that their own inner negative parent is making them feel like an "under dog" and driving them to undermine others instead. Detached people think, "It's no use, everything stinks anyway, so why bother," (see Personality Chart) or desperately trying to bolster their inner feelings of being weak and worthless with megalomania and dreams of greatness.

It is not generally recognized that the human mind tends to play and replay "inner records" that repeat the programming which hostile parent and teacher figures have fed into the mental computer during childhood. Though sometimes well intended, the results are nonetheless damaging. Some common records that play in the neurotic mind are, "I'm no good," "Nothing's any good," "I'll never be able to . . . ," "I'll always fail at . . . ," "Nothing good can happen," "I can't live without . . . ," "I can't stand . . ."—extreme and irrational thoughts which indicate the usurping influence of the negative parents inside the neurotic mind.

Many writers of psychology and religion have pointed out the destructive power of negative thinking and the creative power of positive thinking. Marcus Aurelius wrote, "Very little is needed to make a happy life; it is all within yourself, in your way of thinking." There is truth in this wisdom, but thinking is only one aspect of the human being. The way one thinks is related to and affected by the way one feels. Thoughts and feelings are connected with physical health. The more disturbed one is, the less aware one is of one's "unconscious" mental processes and attitudes. The Self is much more than one's thinking: Unless positive thoughts are sincere, they are illusions. For example, the "nice" neurotic who tries to think and act positively as a way of placating others is afraid and hostile inside. Authentic education and therapy (reeducation) must be a total process that involves the whole being—body, emotions, mind, and spirit.

Neurotic people, who are anxious and defensive, will imagine nonexistent danger, perceiving others as threatening (especially when others remind them of damaging aspects of parental figures). Continuing to live in the past, they repeat self-damaging patterns of behavior. For example, a passive man may continue to be attracted to domineering women, like his mother, despite knowing intellectually that this tendency is self-destructive. Or a woman may be attracted to a cold or sadistic man, like her father, hoping in vain that someway she will manage to obtain his love and change him into her ideal.

Neurotic thinking and perception provokes negative attitudes in others; the attitude one may carry from infancy that people are hurtful becomes a self-fulfilling prophecy. Instinctively we react toward pleasure and away from pain. We often are repulsed by negative physical attitudes and by the verbal messages of negative or anxious individuals. Dr.

Ernst Beier points out, "A person can create beneficial or dangerous emotional environments through body movements and tones of voice."[5]

Peace of mind is a rarity in our society. The healthy, rational mind can exist only as part of an organism that is physically healthy and relaxed and emotionally positive, secure, and loving. In such a state, one is centered in one's inner being (not the head) and identifies with one's inner aliveness—the Life Force itself, and not one's ego. Then the mind is merely a tool that is used to solve the problems of life.

The disturbed person identifies with the mind, which is restless, driven, incapable of finding satisfaction and well-being, and lacking in peace in the present moment (which is its only reality). Caught in fearful, tense watchfulness, one is split from one's wholeness. Trapped in egocentricity, one is unable to get back to one's senses and the here and now. In contrast, the healthy mind is free from the past and free from concerns about the future, enjoying the awareness of being one with reality in the here and now.

Remember that all dimensions of your person—physical, emotional, mental, and spiritual—are interrelated and constantly affecting one another. Dr. John Tilden points out that "a suffering body cripples the mind also." Dr. Herbert Shelton stresses that health is a whole way of life which respects the laws of nature: "Nervous and mental so-called diseases . . . are not set apart from the rest of the body. The unity of pathological phenomena is a fact here as elsewhere." Both of these physicians had a wholistic view of the human organism.

---

[5] Ernst Beier, *The Silent Language of Psychotherapy (2nd edition)*, Aldine Pub. Co., N.Y., 1984.

Thus, improvements in your physical health, through physical exercises, will have a positive effect on your mental state, freeing tension and strengthening your positive feelings. Emotional exercises will inevitably improve your state of mind. Positive changes that you make in your thinking will also increase your physical and emotional health. Decreasing stress will free you to act in more satisfying ways and liberate the loving and assertive feelings that are necessary for self-esteem and happiness.

Now let us move on to examine the defenses we developed in childhood and then Syntonic methods of freeing ourselves from them.

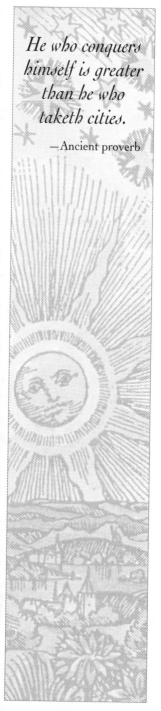

He who conquers himself is greater than he who taketh cities.

—Ancient proverb

T E N

Overcoming Self-Defeating Thoughts and Attitudes

When patients complain to me that it is difficult to free themselves from old patterns and easy to slip back into their former habits, I agree. But I also believe that it is even more difficult to remain the same. Keeping our "safe" yet self-defeating patterns wastes enormous amounts of energy and sabotages the joy and vitality that is our birthright. It is easier to sit at the bottom of a mountain than to climb it. But one never grows in strength, nor does one enjoy the exhilaration of

171

scaling the heights and viewing greater vistas. Gazing up at the mountain is safe and passive, but climbing it is challenging and exciting. When you see your problems as opportunities for growth rather than as obstacles, you are on the way to health.

Having begun this program with the detoxification of your body and the freeing of your energy from rigidity and tension (as outlined in Chapter 3), and having practiced the release exercises to start eliminating negative emotions, you are now ready to corral the positive energy necessary to conquer the neurotic thoughts that sabotage your health and happiness. It is easier to confront the tricky games of your mind after you have mobilized some aggressive energy and feel more of your strength and rage to live.

The Nine Most Common Character Defenses

On the Personality Chart (page xxvii), look at the nine defenses (shown in the second circle from the center). Write each one down, and next to it, as honestly as you can, decide whether it is one of your patterns. Remember that these are all false attitudes, adopted to cover up your real emotions. Most of us had to develop a facade, and now our facade controls us.

1. Deceit

Begin at the top of the chart. Do you tend to be open and honest, or deceitful and devious with others? Humans are the only creature who can feel one way and act another. Most of us had to become more or less deceitful to survive, so if you deny that this is a tendency in yourself, you are more than likely deceiving yourself at this very moment. We also live in a society in which production for profit rather than for the satisfaction of genuine human needs forces people to do things they know are not right. A recent television news story revealed that an international corporation informed the mothers of certain Third World countries that human milk was nutritionally inferior to canned formulas. Obviously this profit-making deceit was damaging to the health of countless babies in the Third World.

Next to your answer, write the way in which you needed to be devious to your family in childhood, out of fear or guilt. Remember, you can love and respect the good aspects of your parents and at the same time be angry at those parts of them that hurt you. The qualities in them which you still resent or hate you will also find in yourself (for example, tendencies to be prudish, irritable, pretentious, perfectionistic, fearful, worrisome, arrogant, or domineering). The more clearly you see these attitudes as parts of yourself that prevent you from feeling free, the more you can make them a target for your positive anger, and thus overcome them gradually. With self-acceptance and respect, you will be able to understand and forgive your parents rather than waste your energy blaming them.

How Hal Regained His Self-Respect

Hal was one of the most deceitful people I'd met in over thirty years of private practice. He had good reason to be. His paranoid father took out his rage against Hal and was jealous of closeness between Hal and his mother, who was as insecure as she was clever. Hal's mother used Hal's fear of his father to manipulate him for her own needs.

Naturally, Hal could not trust anyone, and his whole manner reminded me of that arch symbol of deceit, fear, and distrust—

the devil. Hal's back and shoulders were hunched, his eyes darted here and there, he was always ready to run or attack, he was constantly worrying and scheming, and he totally lacked faith in God, humans, and of course, himself. Having suffered enough, Hal committed himself to Syntonic therapy. His will to live surfaced, and he began to use his brilliant mind, boundless energy, and physical strength *for* rather than against himself.

He fasted to rid his body of excess weight and toxins. He improved his diet and, along with exercising, worked between sessions using Syntonic techniques. Hal learned to use his pent-up rage against his inner enemies. In freeing his mind and body of crippling distortions, he developed the ability to be forthright, open, and honest. He overcame a fear of his own strength (a basic fear in every neurotic person) by learning to direct his rage toward self-liberation rather than against himself and others.

Hal's attitudes changed into more positive ones as he became assertive and productive as a husband, a doctor, and a man with self-respect.

2. Niceness

Do you tend to don a nice front to make others like you, out of insecurity and lack of self-respect? Many of us were taught to "be nice" despite times of real sadness, hurt, and anger. "Niceness" is not to be confused with genuine kindness, which comes from feelings of love, compassion, and consideration for others. In a healthy state, we have genuine self-respect and do not require that others like us; nor do we fear their rejection. Like deceit, false niceness stems from fear.

If you must have others accept you, and if you find it difficult or impossible to say no or to disagree with someone's opinions or beliefs, this is an area in which you are wasting energy. This was once a defense of my own until I overcame the fear that kept me overconcerned with the opinions about me that other people held. This fear was part of the writer's block that I had to struggle against.

If this is in your bag of neurotic defenses, write down the way in which you developed it. Perhaps you learned it from your parents. Challenge the thought, "I must make others like me." In the emotional release exercises, mobilize your anger to overcome this manifestation of fear. Are you constantly anxious when with other people? Do you cultivate this fear even when you are alone, worrying about past or future social situations?

Using the release exercises of yelling, pounding, kicking, and stamping out your anxiety, you will begin to like yourself and others, gradually becoming assertive and positive. And of course, as you grow freer and warmer, others will like you more. When some do not, you will understand that that is *their* problem! Since they do not like themselves, they are not yet capable of liking you. Instead of your old false niceness hiding the hurt and anger deep inside, you will feel compassion and be thankful that you are beginning to enjoy your true inner Self.

How Jill Became Free of Her Inner Child

Jill was a "nice" person who had a desperate fear of not being liked and a constant need to please others no matter what hardships it placed on herself. This pattern, typically, derived from childhood. Jill's father had not wanted a ninth mouth to feed. Her mother had kept her as a "little doll" and could not accept her daughter's need to grow up as a self-assertive adult.

Jill's "niceness" carried over into every aspect of her life. Sexually exploited by some of her employers, she was used as a sex object and a scapegoat. In Syntonic therapy, she understood her plight as I explained her problem using the Personality Chart. A drawing she made of herself as a shapeless wisp further convinced her that she had to struggle to regain and strengthen her essential, real Self.

Jill was able to feel her fear and to cry out her pain, but she had to struggle, with my encouragement, to feel her buried rage. Her rage was so murderous that she had good reason to be afraid of it! I assured her that it was a positive force, if directed against the parts of herself incorporated from her parents and siblings. As she kicked out her fear and "niceness," and pounded into pulp the destructive aspects of her inner "family" images, she discovered that by going deeply enough she could find the clear-flowing stream of life energy, no matter how deeply hidden.

Jill continues to "pull the weeds" in herself when necessary and to "cultivate the flowers" using positive imagery (which will be described in the final section of this book, "The Human Spirit"). She has become one of the warmest, most lovable, compassionate, and assertive human beings I know, and a friend I value greatly.

3. Toughness

Do you tend to have a hard facade instead of a relaxed and friendly one? The tough facade that says "me first" and "I don't care what people think of me" is also a cover-up for fear. As the saying goes, "Every hard-boiled egg is yellow in the middle." If you have this defense, you must have been very hurt in your early life, when these defenses were constructed.

Part of a rigid and tough muscular and character armor, this attitude expresses, "I'm not going to let anyone hurt me again." Like a medieval suit of armor, it prevents one from being hurt, but it also keeps one from feeling pleasure, joy, and love. Examine in which period of your life you developed this armor, and which of your parents you needed it for. Since we often learn these attitudes by example and imitation, chances are that you adopted the very attitude that you feared and hated in some important person in your formative years.

Write down these connections so you can see them clearly in front of you. Understand that this toughness was necessary *then* and that it is a liability *now*. You will come to regard this facade as an inner enemy, a pretense, to be eliminated along with the accompanying secret feelings of loneliness and emptiness. You may discover guilt feelings, because deep down you know you are denying real desires for closeness, warmth, tenderness, and love. As you challenge this attitude and the thoughts, tensions, and fears that go with it, you will begin to feel real strength from your healthy, assertive, and loving Self that has been buried.

How Jim Got Rid of False Toughness

Jim had this kind of "macho" toughness and began to understand that it resulted from the remaining frightened little boy beneath that big, muscular facade which he had built up for protection. Even his handshake was an attack of crushing aggression. In Syntonic therapy, he learned to accept and feel the fear he was hiding by making sounds of fear (into a rolled-up towel for soundproofing). This began to free his breathing and brought into awareness buried memories of painful experiences, which reached back even to a traumatic birth. As his tensions and frozen fear started to thaw, he began to feel the rage that he had locked up in his suit of muscular armor.

He also worked with himself between sessions, and used his rage productively. As he raged against his tough coldness (associated with his stern mother) and his inner weakness (associated with his alcoholic father), and began to feel his sadness, loneliness, and longing for love and closeness. As his body relaxed, he began to feel the flow of positive, assertive, and loving feelings that had been dammed up.

At present, Jim is able to be his own therapist and continue his growth as a more secure, relaxed, reasonable, productive, genuinely sexual, and outgoing human being.

4. Passivity

Do you have a tendency to give up and just wait until things happen? Do you wait for others to initiate events and then follow along, needing their support and hoping for their approval? Do you tend to tell yourself "It's no use" or "I can't win anyway?" Write down the source of this pattern. Remember when you learned to react this way and from whom you learned it.

Part of the process of changing this pattern is to remind yourself constantly, "nothing ventured, nothing gained" and that no one, not even the most powerful and brilliant person you can imagine, can succeed all the time. Some therapies hope that by examining the past and understanding how one's present belief system developed and constantly working to change these beliefs, change can take place. While this has some truth to it, it is only part of the answer.

In the total or wholistic view, other energies and resources can be tapped. Not only can you analyze yourself and think about the source of your passivity (or any other neurotic, self-defeating habit), you can also learn to feel physical tensions that are part of it and mobilize the power within that wants to be free of it. In a passive state you tend toward slumping, lacking backbone, and retreating to the oral-receptive stage of babyhood by putting a cigarette, alcohol or excess food into your mouth.

Such deeply ingrained habits take great effort to change. But the ensuing joy, freedom, productivity, and self-respect are worth hard work. So remind yourself why passivity is a barrier to success and happiness, instead of programming yourself negatively by saying, "I have no willpower." List all the desirable aspects you can think of for breaking this habit. Mobilize your energy and your breathing by lying down and bringing your knees up to your chest. Kick straight out as you exhale, feeling yourself kick out the fear and tension that make you passive. Say along with this action, "I'm tired of being afraid," "I'm sick of blocking myself," and add any other thoughts of this nature. Kick the habit!

Stand up straight and firmly "put your foot down." I use several foam cushions for myself and my patients. Say what you want to do as you stamp. For example, "I *will* finish that work," I *will* make that call" "I *will* be my real Self." You will be picturing yourself as you really are, free of the old doubts, fears, and self-defeating conditioning. In doing so, you are integrating your mind, body, emotions, and the Life Force of the universe in a harmonious and Syntonic way. This is what it means to be whole, together, and integrated.

Jane Finally Put Her Foot Down

Jane had a passivity problem, as many do at times. She traveled a great deal and made herself anxious and tense about packing, incessantly worrying about forgetting things. She tended to avoid the task of packing and would start smoking to allay her anxiety, although she knew this was aggravating a chronic cough and ruining her lungs. Using Syntonic therapy, she conquered *both* her passivity about packing and the smoking habit with my guidance.

In about twelve sessions, Jane had made remarkable progress. For years she had tried a bit of this or that technique for personal change. She had attempted conventional therapy, meditation, hypnosis, self-analysis, and courses in depth psychology. As she put it, however, "I never got things together." The beauty of Syntonic therapy is that all four dimensions of the person are worked with and integrated. "In unity there is strength."

Jane was well motivated. She had already had surgery for smoke- damaged vocal chords and knew her body was declining. And she was sick to death of her attitude of resignation, her endlessly worrying mind, and her spiritual poverty. She fasted and then changed her diet. Healing her hypoglycemia helped her become more calm and quit smoking. She also used the reflexology I taught her how to work on her feet and hands to help the flow of the Life Force to her tired glands and organs.

Jane surprised herself with her rage to live and quickly stamped out her tendencies to say "it's no use" (which, as the weakling in her family, she had developed). She said, "I'm sitting up and standing up like a person and I'm starting to enjoy tackling things I used to dread facing." Her inner mother and sister images took a beating as she "told them off" in her sessions. Her mother and sisters were actually in South America, but to Jane they represented, during sessions, the self-beating parts of herself that had to be cut out like tumorous psychological growths. She began to sleep well and wake up feeling alive and grateful for the gift of another day, free of any self-poisoning drugs.

During group therapy sessions, Jane inspired others with the courage and creative rage with which she challenged her fears and clever rationalizations. She taught others by example that one gains only in proportion to the risks one takes, and between sessions at home she used my cassette tape and continued self-therapy with her body, emotions, mind and Spirit. After only several weeks of therapy, her growth was so marked that people at work were amazed by her new vital way of being. Jane sent others for Syntonic therapy who were ready to take responsibility for their own health and well-being. But best of all, she began to experience what it means to be vital, alive, hopeful, and grateful for the gift of life.

5. Pretended Happiness

The happy front or gay facade is a way of trying to convince the world and oneself that one is not really frightened and sad and angry. But, as Ohsawa, a Zen master with whom I once studied would say, "The bigger the front, the bigger the back."

People with this predominant defense often were the family or classroom clowns. They often become entertainers and comedians and are always "on." This actually means that they are always on edge, afraid that someone might get through to their inner feelings. They are constantly the life of the party and attempt to make others believe that they're really cool and have life by the tail.

Alone with themselves, however, it is a different story. No longer performing, they are faced with their actual anxiety and confusion. Unable to feel comfortable with themselves and lacking the support and approval of others, they become depressed and lonely. Often such people turn to compulsive eating, drinking, sex, smoking, or drug taking. This never successfully eases their deep feelings of loneliness and worthlessness. They are driven to continue their charade with the outside world until they exhaust themselves and withdraw once again. There is no way out of this manic-depressive cycle unless one is able to find help to face and overcome the terror, rage, and despair that lurk within.

Do you tend to put on a cheerful front and not even let
your friends know that at times you feel depressed, frightened, or discouraged? Ask yourself what is the worst thing
that would happen if you were more honest with friends.
Write down the reasons for this pretense—when you
started it and whom you were imitating or perhaps placating. Then ask yourself if it is worth the price you pay for it
now (your health, relationships, and self-respect). If you
wish to break free of this pattern, it will take a struggle. The
more entrenched a bad habit, and the more "satisfaction"
you get from it, the harder it is to change. Remember, you
have within you God-given intelligence, physical strength,
emotional power, and the Life Force. If you put all of these
together, they will be far stronger than the facade you had
to erect and that now demands of you constant mortgage
payments and endless repairs. If you are ready to free yourself, this total syntonic method is all you need, provided that
you are honest with yourself.

Ned—From Cool to Real

Ned was a cool character, a sharp dresser, always had a joke
for every occasion and used pot and cocaine occasionally. He
was not one to turn down a good deal, even if others would get
hurt by it. He had no guilt feelings that he was aware of to stand
in his way.

His father had been a successful hustler, and although there
was much that Ned hated about his father, he was just like him:
brash, self-centered, vain, pretentious, and cold. Ned felt both
pity and hostility for his mother, a weak and anxious woman
who had used Ned for the emotional warmth that was lacking in
her husband.

Ned came for help after a friend, who had been successful in

Syntonic therapy, convinced him that his drug trip was heading for the rocks. Ned had been in two other more conventional therapies, and this was his last try. I showed him the Personality Chart and asked him to pick out the parts that fit his character. He identified a number of defenses but grinned as he picked out the characteristic "I'm so cool." He also saw many of his symptoms in the outside ring, but he became serious for the first time when I told him that the way to the center meant going through the inner hell he had spent most of his life denying.

Ned had a long struggle between the devil (his clever and frightened inner child) and the deep blue sea (his longing for peace and wholeness). So he struggled, ran away, and returned to struggle some more. He was able to mobilize some anger and make some progress against his inner fears, but he was most afraid of softening enough to feel the deep pain and sadness at never having been genuinely loved and cared for. His third marriage had collapsed, and he was once again alone with himself. Acute sadness broke the dam, and gradually his deeper rage started to flow. He had glimpsed it before in wild explosions, but this time he learned to channel it and direct it at the parts of himself that he would no longer tolerate. Instead of being proud of his psychopathic operations, he now saw them as part of the fearful, clever child within, rather than as a part of himself.

Gradually his posture changed; his face softened; his eyes changed from black pools to clear blue; and his hands and feet were no longer cold and sweaty. He had kicked the drug habit, as well as the cool facade and the conman approach to life that was actually a way of death for him. He was on the way to becoming a real man—a person he could like and live with.

6. Contempt

If nothing is any good, then there is nothing to want, nothing to risk, and nothing to regret. This defense of denial is one of the most difficult to overcome. One makes a pact with the devil, as it were, and sells one's soul for an absolute guarantee of impregnable safety. The reverse side of this contract, however, in very small print, makes it clear that faith, hope, and love, in any form, are to be strictly avoided.

Oscar Wilde described this facade in one of his clever sayings, "One can't exaggerate the unimportance of anything." But even Dorian Gray looked into the mirror one day and saw the specter before his eyes. This pattern is one of slow suicide through rampant overindulgence. Rarely does one escape disaster. The hapless person caught in this web gets meager satisfaction from putting everything down. The trouble is that he or she is *part* of everything and is *also* an object of contempt underneath a vain pretense of superiority.

If contempt is your self-protective mechanism, the same principles hold; to face your problem and create a strategy to overcome it. You will be motivated to make an effort to save yourself if, at the end of your rope, failure, despair, or intense fear push you into action. Again, write down when you decided on this course, in relation to which people in your past, and under what circumstances. You will need more positive energy than you will be able to muster within yourself to overcome this pattern, so try to realize that asking a therapist or a Higher Power for help is the most important step you can make.

Anger, if used against the parts of yourself you hate (instead of against life, others, and yourself), can be a tremendous positive force. Remember that deep down your real Self is there, however long it has been buried and denied.

How Carmen Got Rid of Contempt

Carmen had this attitude, and with good reason. She had been the unfortunate child of a very disturbed mother, who had been a prostitute and encouraged her daughter to follow in her footsteps from the age of twelve. Carmen was afraid of her mother's violence after alcoholic binges and dared not oppose her wishes. She had never known her father, but she learned that she could manipulate men and use sex as an instrument of her contempt for them. She became a prostitute who "specialized" in whipping men who "enjoyed" being beaten and were suffering from self-contempt.

Driven by unbearable physical, mental, and emotional pain and a terror of losing control and going crazy, Carmen sought psychiatric help. She was given drugs to deaden her pain, but they left her depressed and exhausted. What kept her going was a hope of someday becoming an actress (the only joy in her childhood had been when she had been taken to see films). In her fantasies, Carmen pictured herself as a beautiful heroine who was able to overcome all obstacles and eventually find happiness.

In Syntonic therapy, Carmen realized that neither drugs nor talking endlessly about her problems was the answer. She understood that freeing her energy had to be a total process, involving all parts of herself. She changed her way of eating after a cleansing fast and got more rest and exercise. She was encouraged to express all her feelings by connecting them with sounds and movements. Gradually her deep sadness melted the tensions in her body and strengthened her rage to live.

Carmen learned gradually to direct her wild explosiveness against the parts of herself that she hated and the images of people from her tragic life that she still carried within. She realized that her contemptuous attitude and the negative "records" she constantly played in her mind had been programmed by others. She saw that others had used her as a scapegoat for their hostility and contempt, and that she had accepted this mistreatment.

The turning point in growth inevitably comes when one distinguishes between one's defenses and one's real Self. Then a target for one's hostility is recognized, and a way out of the web of inner energy-wasting conflicts is possible.

Turning her rage against the tensions, fears, and negative thoughts that obsessed her life, Carmen began to feel free and relaxed for the first time in her life. She also worked with herself between sessions, speeding up the process of change tremendously. At the end of each session, I taught Carmen the technique of positive imagery and cosmic mediation described in Chapter 14. Carmen's contempt, like all defenses, was a symptom of fear, tension, and negative thinking that blocked the natural flow of energy. The more free, relaxed, and alive she became, the more she enjoyed and valued herself and living.

7. Detachment

The pattern of detachment is the neurotic orientation par excellence. It is dedicated to safety at all costs. Dominated by fear, one prevents oneself from accepting the fact that life is a gamble, and one is dedicated to the belief that one is "better safe than sorry." While it is wise and necessary to exercise some caution in life, to let caution subvert courage and risk taking is self-crippling.

If this is one of your inclinations, you will realize how often you have been angry at yourself for letting opportunities slip by that would have resulted in positive growth and benefits for your life. Which part of yourself is endlessly reminding you to hold back and never be spontaneous? As children, we frequently absorb the anxieties of one or both parents and carry their "records" within ourselves for the rest of our lives.

Examine this pattern by writing down the sources of your fear. List the differences between realistic carefulness and the fearfulness that can keep you alone, timid, frustrated, and always sitting the game out on the bench. Somewhere you are angry at this constant self-denial which you inflict on yourself in the name of "reason." Accept this anger as a good and positive force—if used constructively—to help you overcome your obsession with being safe. Turn your anger on the fear (blocked energy), tension, and childish thinking that you maintain.

Spend several minutes every morning challenging this pattern. Through release exercises you can kick out, pound out, and stamp out this archaic habit by unifying your physical, emotional, and mental energies. This wholistic system will conquer any undesirable pattern when you have decided that you have had enough of it. When you combine the *will* to change with the *power* to energize your thinking, you will then have the *willpower* to accomplish your purpose. Without this power, all the thought in the world is mere abstraction. And without the thought to guide it, all the power you possess is scattered and useless.

I remember Plato's description of this condition in the allegory of the charioteer from a course in philosophy. The mind is represented by the charioteer, the body is like the chariot, and the emotional energies that supply the power are like the horses. One without the other is useless at best and disastrous at worst. The secret is releasing and channeling energy for constructive purposes. For this reason, wholistic techniques are far more effective than working with or stressing one part of the person, whether it be the body, the emotions, the mind, or the spirit. They are all necessary and essential parts of the whole!

So if you want to break through your past conditioning, get your emotions together with your body and your head. The more diligently you work on overcoming your fearful detachment, the more you will succeed. After each workout with yourself, picture in your mind the way you want to be. These mental rehearsals will water the seeds of your real Self to grow, after a long hibernation of "safety." Energy follows thought, and after a release and self-assertive session you will have far greater energy available to redirect.

Allow yourself, in this positive fantasy, to approve of being your free, outgoing, and true Self. But remember, positive fantasy must be followed by *new action* and *behavior* in your real life. Haven't you wasted enough energy in grandiose fantasies about being the all-conquering hero, while remaining Ms. or Mr. Milquetoast in your daily life?

How Glenn Stopped Blaming and Started Living

Glenn had a serious case of detachment. He had been the shy and sickly only child of overanxious parents who were preoccupied with what the neighbors would think and always worried about the dangers of living. Glenn was not allowed to learn gradual independence but was constantly supervised and regarded as a sickly child, even as an adolescent.

He was programmed to feel constantly anxious and to think the worst of any available situation. Worrying constantly about all the negative possibilities leads to detached withdrawal from life. Repeating his parents' example, Glenn never stopped worrying. Although a bright boy, he worried so much about exams in school that his mind would go blank. Instead of facing the situation at hand, he would start his record of saying "what if" this and "what if" that and dream up paralyzing fears.

Although he grew to be a well-built young man, Glenn thought of himself as weak and sickly and was always afraid that he could not cope with life. He tended to withdraw into a dream world, where he was strong and powerful and possessed great sexual prowess and financial success—"Then they will know I'm somebody and want my company, and I'll be on top of the pile." As an overprotected child who never had the right to express his feelings and thoughts within his family, Glenn had lost touch with his inner Self and his sense of self-respect.

To compensate for his loneliness and to relieve his inner anxiety about losng his job as an engineer, Glenn headed for bars after work. The alcohol temporarily deadened his inner stress, and the company of other lonely drinkers kept him from the even more unbearable loneliness of being in his own company at home. As he became overweight and his health declined, his physician suggested that Glenn seek therapeutic help.

Underneath his feeble attempts to please and amuse, Glenn was very anxious and bitter. His fantasies about his associates were at times murderously hostile. I assured Glenn that he had valid reasons to feel frightened, sad, and furious, and I showed him the Personality Chart. He recognized detachment as his main defensive characteristic, along with several others. He found it hopeful and reassuring that there was a real Self underneath. He said, "If that's there, I'm going to find it. Nothing else has worked anyway."

Motivated by a desire to release his pain, overcome his drinking addiction, and find the wellness that I emphasized was his birthright, Glenn got to work. His clever inner child tried to resist his growth every step of the way. But Glenn quickly learned that his inner rage could be used as a positive force for growth. He fasted for a few days to lose weight and detoxify his body. The discovery that he had the capacity for self-discipline boosted his self-esteem. He began to exercise, joined a sports group, and began to practice being honest with people about his feelings, whenever possible.

When he no longer wasted energy blaming his parents for what they did to him, Glenn faced that now he was responsible for his own life and his own state of health. As he became physically and emotionally stronger, his thinking became more positive and assertive. He began to realize that his suffering enabled him to have deep understanding and compassion for other people. In group therapy, he became well-liked and respected for his honesty and his courage in taking risks when using the release exercises in the group. In group therapy, integrating one's body, emotions, and thoughts by pounding and stamping is more helpful than any partial methods of self-expression.

Glenn came a long way from being detached. He found that he could really care about himself and others and decided, with my wholehearted agreement, that he would go back to graduate studies and later train to become a Syntonic therapist.

8. False Pride

Setting ourselves up (in fantasy or behavior) as a superior being is something we do when we lose touch with our essence or real Self. Through inner fear and tension, we adopt neurotic strategies as defenses of the ego system. When out of tune with life and out of harmony with ourselves, we may at times employ any of these mental tricks. Our thoughts twist reality with self-destructive cleverness, in a vain attempt to avoid the pain of inner conflicts and anxious tenson. We have lost our wholeness, and our thoughts are no longer in harmony with our true Self. William Butler Yeats wrote,

> God, guard me from the thoughts
> Men think in the mind alone,
> He who sings a happy song,
> Thinks in a marrow bone.

Only when we are in a state of wholeness are our thoughts connected with our true nature, and only then do they evince a true expression of our authentic Self.

Aristotle knew the state of positive being I call the Self and suggested that if a person has one genuine virtue—courage, diligence, honesty, or humility—he or she has them all. But we finite human beings can slip from our true center and get caught up in the clever games of the ego. Some people's central defense becomes pride and, driven by inner feelings of inadequacy and inferiority, they set themselves up as being better than anyone else.

The first chapter of this book discussed the perceptive terminology of body language and folk wisdom. We speak of "stiff-necked pride" and of a haughty attitude as a person "above it all." Unlike those who carry a resigned and defeated posture, those with prideful defense show their arrogance in their stiff posture. But they are not grounded in reality, and they get carried away with their conceit. Sooner or later their inability to see reality and their desperate drive to be superior lead to self-destruction. Hence, the wisdom of the proverb "Pride goeth before a fall."

If you have this defense character trait, it will take work and courage to face and overcome it. As with other defenses, we usually only relinquish it when it has caused us more pain than it is worth. If you have a constant need to tell yourself and be told by others how great you are, take a moment to ask yourself why you feel so worthless. Take an objective look at your life, and see how you developed this attitude. If you can admit that you are insecure and tense inside and wish to change this unhappy condition, you can start now to outgrow your infantile grandiosity.

Look objectively at your life and find out how you developed this false pride. Often it begins when one has been constantly rewarded by one or both parents for being better than others, or has been overpraised for achievements and constantly reminded that one is better than this or that person or group. It is often the result of a spoiled-child pattern, in which the inner child, who never received necessary discipline and limitations, continues to act out this narcissistic pattern as an adult.

Underneath, the spoiled child always feels unloved and senses that he or she is being used for the satisfaction of the parents. Afraid of the child's anger or rejection and needing the child's love because they lack self-acceptance, such parents are unable to set sensible limits for the child. Likewise, their values are always in terms of outer show and success and never in terms of inner growth and true well-being.

To free yourself, first you must get in touch with your inner tension, fear, and sadness. You will feel relief when you let go of these inner feelings through the language of emotion. The hostility that you express by putting others down is turned against yourself when you fail to be the best in everything. List the assets and liabilities of this attitude and ask yourself, "Would I need this attitude if I were in touch with my real Self?" We have all glimpsed the center of our being. If this is the way you really want to be—and that is the way that brings peace of mind—you are ready to begin to free yourself.

Challenge this false part of you and see it as separate from yourself. Rather than constantly holding onto it, see it as an enemy that wastes your energy, undermines your authentic self-respect, and alienates others. Mobilize your physical strength and your anger, and use the release exercises to challenge your vanity.

After you kick, pound, and stamp out this part of yourself and the images of people who twisted your personality in this way, focus on relaxing your neck. If it is still stiff, tighten it as you inhale, hold for a count of three, and release the tension as you exhale sharply. The more your neck relaxes and your breathing deepens into your abdomen, the more you will begin to feel your center, below your navel.

As you relax and become more centered, you will feel more secure. The more secure you feel, the more clearly you will think. Thinking clearly, you will accept that you are a finite human being and no longer have to "strut and fret your brief hour" on the stage of life as Shakespeare so beautifully wrote.

Karen Finds Her Inner Beauty

Karen had been the little darling of her family and was much younger than her brothers and sisters. Constantly fussed over and played with, she never had the chance to be with herself and to learn things on her own. She quickly learned to exploit her exploiters and manipulated them into helping her with her school homework and writing term papers for her. A pretty child, she was nicknamed "Beauty" and became obsessed with the way she looked. So great was her preoccupation with outer things that she would change her clothes several times a day and hate to wear anything more than once. She thought she was the most perfect and wonderful person ever, but of course was always concerned that someone else might be prettier and better dressed.

Karen's feelings, however, were far different from her blown-up self-image. True, she was stunning and a successful model, but she did not *feel* beautiful because she had ugly and conflicted feelings inside. Her beautiful facade was a cover-up for a Pandora's box of negativity. Never having felt loved and respected for being herself, she had no real self-confidence. Living only in her head and feeling tense and frigid among others, she felt that her life was going by without real friendships and love. Beneath her carefully made-up facade was tremendous hostility, as with every other person whose real needs were not respected during childhood. Spiritually cut off from any connection with the source of her being, Karen was a belligerent atheist, like all prisoners of false pride.

But defenses crumble sooner or later, since they are false constructions. This is when people seek help. Without such growing pains, one would never search for reality or have the opportunity to change. As Karen approached her middle twenties, she began to lose her pseudoconfidence and worry about younger models taking her place. Since her inner resources were so totally undeveloped, an extra pound of weight or a slight wrinkle was a harbinger of disaster to her. Karen literally began to shake before the camera, and began to use drugs and alcohol to control her fears. Aware that she needed help, she struggled to discover the inner maturity that was so lacking in her life.

At first, afraid to let down her hair, she wanted merely to talk superficially about her problems. But I convinced her that this would take years and perhaps never help her. She realized from the Personality Chart that her facade had been built to hide the painful feelings that accompanied her role as the "little doll" of her family. She finally dared to risk the expression of sounds and movements, and she discovered that she had a "black ball" inside that was always there (i.e., fear). Each time she cried or connected with her feelings of rage, this black ball of fear became smaller.

Gradually Karen was no longer worried about who might see her leave a session with her hair in disarray. She began to realize how much she hated her nickname "Beauty" and the people who gave it to her. As is always the case in genuine emotional growth, Karen's rage helped her conquer her inner fears and bodily tensions. As she became more relaxed, her positive feelings could finally begin to flow. She no longer needed to worry about others, and the envy which had corroded her being melted away. When she began to feel like a beautiful person within and could love herself and others, her false pride disappeared.

Occasionally in a profound process such as Syntonic therapy, certain patterns and beliefs may be traced back before birth. Sometimes when people feel their "stuckness" on a very deep level, they perceive that they are caught inside by something that will not let them go. Our culture so often fights and denies the natural order that even the birth process may become an unnecessarily traumatic and drug-laden experience.

In Karen's case, she experienced her Self as curled up inside her mother and not wanting to be born, sensing in some way that she had not been a wanted child. This was in fact partly true, for Karen was eighteen years younger than her next sibling. She discovered that every morning she would wake up with this same attitude: fists clenched, body tense, and not wanting to go out and face the day. After she had a rebirth experience in her therapy session, Karen began to awaken relaxed and ready to enjoy the challenge of another day.

9. Spite

Spite is an intense form of masochism, a method of turning one's anger against oneself, of "cutting off your nose to spite your face." As in all neurotic mechanisms, there is also a method to this madness. Its purpose is to retaliate against and hurt those who have hurt oneself while secretly enjoying the safety of one's own misery. As with all deep character traits, it begins early in childhood. While it has strong elements of passivity, contempt, detachment, and deceit, the fundamental process of spite is the desire to hurt others by hurting oneself. Usually this pattern develops in children who have been both cruelly treated and constantly controlled. Their fear is stronger than their rage, and consequently they tend to act out their anger against themselves. Actually, they are playing against themselves the roles of negative parents and are too afraid to oppose their oppressors.

Prey to this conditioning, one becomes one's own worst enemy. Under the rubric of "I don't care," the spiteful person sabotages himself or herself at every turn, afraid to take the risks of living and instead championing self-defeat with the thought that "they'll be sorry." "They," of course, could be dead and buried, but this deeply conditioned pattern can continue nonetheless. The inner tragic drama plays on, even though there is no audience in the theater.

Do you find that you often sabotage the goals you tell yourself you want to achieve? Do you provoke people to reject you and then tell yourself you don't care? Do you deny yourself the pleasure of relaxing and enjoying things — the pleasures of eating, playing, love making, socializing, and experiencing spiritual joyfulness? Do you find that everything seems to go wrong and then shrug as if it doesn't matter anyway? Do you get secret satisfaction out of being a martyr and having the worst fate of anyone you know?

Dostoyevsky began one of his profoundly self-searching novels *Notes From the Underground*, thus: "I am a sick man. I am a spiteful man." This is an expression of the self-destructive use of one's energy as a form of illness. To be spiteful is to be caught in one of the circles of hell from which it is not easy to extricate oneself.

First look at yourself and decide whether you are getting back at others by hurting yourself. Perhaps you will remember times in your childhood when you denied yourself things you wanted as a kind of self-punishment. Afraid to care about yourself, your growth, and your happiness, do you subtly try to protect yourself from any risk taking? Also recognize your anger. Although there may be valid reasons for feeling anger (we are all the products of our conditioning), admit that hurting yourself is a tragic way of express-ing your hostility. It will be helpful to write down the pros and cons of your spitefulness. Take an objective look at the inner child you have been allowing to run your life. The fact is you do care—and your secret fantasies of the good things of life prove it.

Once you perceive the root of this pattern and under-stand how twisted is the satisfaction you receive from it, you will be ready to challenge that neurotic part which you wish to overcome by means of combining your physical and emo-tional strength with your willpower. You will then be able to rechannel the energy you have misused, by releasing ten-sions, fears, and negative thoughts and images from within—and you will be on the road to freedom (see 15 Steps, p. 151).

Growth is a fluctuating process, like the tacking of a sail-boat. Moment by moment one goes as far as possible and then swings back to safety before going on to risk greater progress. If the going is too tough and you need more help, find a therapist or group which incorporates the mind, body, and emotions as equals and in which you will have guidance toward regaining your spiritual awareness and oneness with the Life Force that created you. This power is always there when you learn to open yourself to it!

Seven Points to Remember in Dealing with Your Self-damaging and Neurotic Attitudes

- The nine major neurotic attitudes are deceit, nice-ness, toughness, passivity, pretended happiness or gaiety, contempt, detachment, false pride, and spite.

- The more tension and fear we experienced in childhood, the more these defenses were needed.
- Though they served a purpose then, now they are self-defeating and block all aspects of our growth.
- To free yourself of them, you must first face the ones you are allowing to exist in your life.
- By owning each pattern, understanding its source, and mobilizing your physical, emotional, and mental energies, each of these crutches can gradually be discarded.
- Since the fear of being real underlies them all, the more you mobilize your rage to live, the more you will overcome your fear.
- The more you develop your "inner kingdom"—that is, feel your center and wholeness—the more loving and assertive you will be. The more you cultivate and experience your real Self, the less you will need neurotic defenses. (See the Personality Chart.)

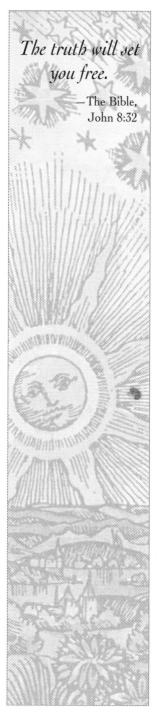

The truth will set you free.

—The Bible, John 8:32

ELEVEN

Syntonic Ways to Free Your Mind

Physical well-being and emotional harmony combined with a clear mind are requisite for a rich, happy, and healthy life. We all know that the way we feel affects the way we think. If we feel physically sick or tired, emotionally down in the mouth, anxious, or destructively angry, we will tend to think discouraging, unreasonable, or negative thoughts.

The opposite is also true! The way we think strongly affects the way we feel! For example, if we think of life as

199

a meaningless accident, we will feel bored and/or cynical. If we think of the beauty of creation in its marvelous order and variety we will realize that life is a precious gift and an exciting adventure.

How To Stop Repeating Negative Programming

Everything that happens to us is imprinted in that fantastic mechanism, the human mind. The imprinting the mind receives from birth stays there throughout life.

After a healthy, natural birth, the infant in its mother's arms is peaceful and trusting. Dr. Leboyer has photographed this happy state, as well as infants who were disturbed by a traumatic birth followed by separation from the mother. The agony of their suffering is the strongest argument I know for nonviolent birthing.[1] Here is the beginning of negative programming starting at birth.

In the early years, the tense, hostile, frightened, or sad words of parents and teachers register in the child's mind and program his or her thinking in damaging and negative ways. The inner kingdom of beauty and order with which we are born often becomes an inner battlefield of pain and confusion. There is a difference between being told "You are a bad girl [boy]" and being told that what you are *doing* is bad or dangerous. Often as children we were condemned for the wrong reasons—for example, when asking honest questions about sex, we were told we had dirty minds; when feeling pleasure in our bodies, we were viewed as bad or wicked; when being open and truthful to our feelings, we were punished for our expressions of fear or anger.

---

[1] Frederick LeBoyer, op. cit. p. 41.

It should give us pause to realize that in training wild and domesticated animals, the best results come from constant gentleness and the rewarding of positive feelings and behavior—never from hurting and frightening the animal. In experimental laboratories, animals are made anxious, disturbed, and neurotic by giving them conflicting signals (such as when food is given along with a shock). Similarly, as children we are often told to tell the truth and then are punished and treated with disrespect when we are, in fact, being honest.

The first part of strengthening our mental health is to become aware of our destructive and unreasonable thoughts. The first thoughts that must be expelled are ones like "I'm no good" and "I'll never be able to do this or that." Sometimes we think such thoughts because we were told as children "You can't do anything right" and "You'll never amount to anything"—which made us feel hurt and hopeless, and undermined both our reverence for life and our self-respect. Such thoughts tend to come to mind—like vultures swarming to a dead animal—when we feel tense and angry, thereby making us more tense, hurt, and angry.

Make a list of the negative "records" you tend to play to yourself. Next to each write a reasonable, assertive thought to counteract the negative thought. Whenever such thoughts come to mind, oppose them with positive and realistic thoughts. Gradually you will cease to put yourself down and will appreciate and respect yourself. If you continue to tell yourself the destructive things you were told in childhood, you will be responsible for your own unhappiness. As Tom Paine wrote as a political leader during the American revolt against England, "the price of freedom is eternal vigilance." The price of *inner* freedom is also vigilance and constructive effort, much like tending a garden. If you passively let the weeds grow (or water and cultivate them!), they will soon choke out your fruits and flowers.

Second, eliminate any perfectionistic ideas which you may use to judge yourself in a cruel and hurtful way. Just as no garden grows entirely free of weeds, there are no perfect people without faults and limitations. We all have strengths and weaknesses. The best athletes strike out, double fault, and fumble. However, they continue to play and learn from their mistakes, rather than curse themselves for being imperfect or defeat themselves by undermining their own confidence.

Exaggerated thoughts must also be corrected because they stir up unnecessary doubts and fears. Many of these, carried over from childhood, derive from the inner child within: "It would be terrible if this or that person didn't like me," "I can't stand being alone," "It's so awful to fail, so I won't try anything," "I'll never be able to do that," "It always works out badly if I'm honest," and "Better safe than sorry."

Beneath fear and hopelessness, there is anger. Irrational, destructive thoughts are connected with physical tension and angry feelings. When we try to defeat the urge to grow (or allow others to do so), a rage to live arises. Instead of turning this rage on ourselves or others, turn this rage on your negative and self-defeating thoughts as well as the unreasonable fears and tensions that accompany them.

To strengthen your *willpower,* try the following exercise. Write down the negative thoughts that you tend to repeat mentally. Then place pillows on the floor, and start putting your foot down, strongly, exhaling sharply each time you do. Stamp with anger at each negative thought on your list. This will integrate your mind, body, and emotions and increase your feeling of syntony and wholeness. Attack each destructive thought and attitude beginning with the words, "I'm tired of . . . ." After you have released some of your anger and hostility in a constructive way, put your foot down in an assertive way with each positive thought and attitude that you wish to strengthen. Begin each assertive expression with the words "I will." Integrating mental, physical, and emotional energies, your thoughts will become more reasonable, constructive, and assertive. They will strengthen your positive emotions and in turn be strengthened by them. An auspicious circle will be established rather than a vicious one, and you will gain not only greater self-respect but also the respect of others.

If cultivating your inner garden seems difficult, remember that staying stuck and not growing only *seems* easier and brings with it frustration and hopelessness. Growing pains can lead to deeper satisfaction and well-being. Our attitudes about life experiences determine whether we stagnate or grow through the problems of living.

Using Adversity Positively

One person may lose a job or fail a test or end a relationship, tell her or himself that this as too terrible to bear, and become an addict, an alcoholic, a dropout, or even attempt suicide. Another may regard the same failure with hostility and/or spite and continue repeating the same mistakes. A third person may *learn* and *grow* through the failure by more positive thinking; "I must learn from this, see what I have to face and change in myself, and make the best of this painful experience." We all have made mistakes and experienced failures and, undoubtedly, will err again. But we can make our biggest problems our *greatest opportunities*. Drop the idea of perfection and make growing your goal. Since life never stands still, accept growing as a star to steer by rather than as a final destination.

Another aspect of mental health is quieting the activity of the mind. Eastern gurus were looking into the inner universe for centuries while Western scientists were exploring the outer universe. In Hinduism there is a saying (which I quoted earlier), "The mind is like a monkey on a tree, endlessly chattering and jumping about." As we learn to quiet this mental chattering (which is related to physical tension and emotional anxiety), we can approach that priceless state called peace of mind, which is described in the Scriptures as "the peace that passeth understanding." This state is beyond thought and understanding, but we can measure its relaxing effect on our bodily functions—blood pressure lowers, the heart beats more slowly, anxiousness lessens, and breathing becomes easier and quieter. You then have the freedom to think or not think.

To find this state of being—to refresh ourselves and quiet our minds for short periods of time each day—is part of the wisdom of living. It requires self-awareness and self-knowledge and practice. "Know Thyself" was spoken by the Oracle of Delphi of Greece and are known as the wisest words ever uttered. We have yet to practice this Greek teaching in our schools and colleges, in which we learn about almost everything *except* the most important thing of all—ourselves. (See Appendix 4 for a fuller treatment of this subject.)

There are different methods of clearing and quieting our minds. Some people use a mantra—a sound or syllable which is kept in one's mind to exclude busy chattering and worrying. In a way, using a mantra is like juggling, because it is difficult to focus your attention on worrisome thoughts while concentrating on the mantra. Another method is to focus awareness on the body and breathing. Try lying or sitting comfortably and, with awareness, breathe gently into the center of your body just below your navel. If thoughts come, observe them. Let them come and go from your mind, and remain aware of your breathing and your center. Gradually thoughts will lose the power to disturb you, and you will learn to control your mind rather than letting your mind control you. You will move out of the darkness of your conditioning toward enlightenment. When your mind becomes your servant rather than your master, you will become free of the cycle of negative, destructive thoughts from your past that are of no real value.

Another technique used to quiet the mind is to remember a time and place when you felt most peaceful in your mind and body. Perhaps it was when you were lying restfully on a beach. Remember the feeling of the warm sand, the smell of the surf, the sound of the seagulls, the taste of the salt water. Picture your mind free of thoughts, like a clear, infinite, cloudless sky.

The more we get "back to our senses," the more free we become from the domination of our minds.

One of the favorite meditative techniques in my morning syntonic tune-up regimen is one that I learned from Dr. Stephen T. Chang.[2] It is from the Taoist tradition of China and is called "beating the heavenly drum." Place your index fingers next to the opening of your ears, and move them so that they press the little flap of your ears into the ear opening. You will hear a sound like a water-fall. Sitting upright and relaxed, ideally in the Zen position sitting back on your heels, tap on the nails of your index fingers with your middle fingers. You may tap from twelve to thirty six times, and repeat for a total of three times.

---

[2] Stephen T. Chang, *The Book of Internal Exercises*, Strawberry Hill Press, San Francisco, Ca., 1978, pp. 56, 57.

When this is done properly you will hear a pleasant vibratory sound like a drumbeat. This is not only healthy for the ear, but also stimulates the pineal gland which in Taoism is the center for spiritual awareness. I experience indescribable calm and serenity after this procedure and find such liberation that I think of it as the gateway to Nirvana, that state in which one is totally free from ego. When I return to the mundane realm, I have a sense of freedom which I wish for you; an ability to remain serene and maintain my Self in almost any circumstance. The sages describe this level of enlightenment as being "in the world but not of it." At long last, one is no longer a chronic victim of the emergency fight or flight anxiety response of the autonomic nervous system.

If you practice these techniques every day, along with healthy nutrition, methods to relax your body, and—when necessary—exercises to release negative emotions, greater peace of mind will be the priceless gift you give yourself.

Eight Keys to Overcoming Negative Thinking

- List the negative thoughts or "records" you play to yourself.
- Next to each one, write reasonable thoughts to counter them.
- If the negative thoughts are stronger, use emotional release techniques to challenge them: Stamping, pounding, and kicking will help you mobilize constructive anger.
- Counter perfectionistic thoughts in the same way.
- Remember the hare and the tortoise: Slow, steady gains are better than spurts followed by discouragement and resignation.

- Keep in mind that the problems of living are opportunities for growth and learning.
    Practice quieting your mind by
    Keeping awareness of the point just below your
       navel.
    Focusing on a mantra or a sound or the word one.
    Focusing on breathing for several minutes at a
       time.
    Imagining a place where you have been most
       serene.
    Beating the heavenly drum.
- Gradually you can learn to make your mind your
  servant, rather than your master.

The Human Spirit

He who sees the oneness under
ten thousand things is ready to return
where he has always been.

—A CHINESE (TAOIST) SAYING

The lord is the spirit and where the
spirit of the lord is there is freedom.

II CORINTHIANS 3:17

TWELVE

How To Have a Dynamic and Positive Spirit

The Sources of Spiritual Sickness

The emotionally healthy and undamaged human being has a dynamic and positive spirit; the life energy flows through a relaxed body freely and expresses itself in a general feeling of love toward oneself, others, and life itself. My friend and teacher, the late Paul Tillich, did not find "God" in some "being" created by the finite mind. He spoke of God *beyond* our conception of God, the very

211

source and ground of Being. For him religion was not ritual or any arbitrary, random "belief," but matters of "ultimate concern." Religion (the word means "to bind together") in the true sense means living with a positive attitude or spirit. The fruits of this attitude are faith, hope, and love.

In this century, neurosis—distrust, despair, and hatred—and technology have brought more destruction of life than ever before. Cynicism about the human spirit and human nature is rampant. In my view, it is not human nature that is at fault. Rather, the fault lies with destructive educational practices from the formative years of life which damage human nature and crush or twist the natural, positive flow of human vitality.

The negative aspect of the human mother is symbolized by traditional depictions of the witch. Dressed in black, with her cruel face and a stick symbolizing destructive aggression, she represents the threatening power of the neurotic, disturbed mother who denies the infant the love and security necessary for the child to remain trusting and whole. This process ruptures the core of love and the natural feeling of being one with life. For it is the flowing energy of love which unifies the personality with itself and with the outer world and creates Syntony.

Fear and anxiety turn humans against themselves and others and separate them from the state of Oneness with God or the Life Force. This spiritual malaise that undermines most cultures makes up the emotional plague of fear and negativity. It has afflicted humankind since the mythical Fall from Grace, when humans' new power of thought enabled them to violate the growth of the personality and the laws of nature.

Wherever the natural function of motherhood is damaged, outweighed by the negative power of the witch, the result is inevitably the development of the negative attitudes in humans symbolized by the image of the devil. Neurosis is not only the fault of the witch; the unloving father also participates in sabotaging the child's self-worth and positive growth. The witch and devil no more exist as objects than do gremlins or angels or gods. But religious and therapeutic psychology, which explores the depths of humans through their dreams and nightmares, reveal that such demonic forces do exist in emotional and spiritual illness. This is illustrated in the following case study.

A patient, whom I shall name Gregory, had become a con man, driven to anxiety and shrewdness by a hurtful upbringing. His mother was alternately withdrawn or angry, and his father unpredictably hostile. Gregory dreamed that he was barricaded in his house against a man and woman who were threatening his life. They represented the negative aspects of his mother and father. Gregory allowed the woman to enter, thinking that he could con her into letting him escape to safety. But she was not trustworthy, and as he realized that she would betray him he awoke in terror. His chronic state of inner fear and tension, his crushed spirit and sense of worthlessness are best described as hell, which Dostoyevsky defined as "the condition of those who cannot love" in *The Brothers Karamazov*. In Syntonic therapy, Gregory was able to gradually release his fear and hatred and destroy these inner negative parental images through visualization and catharsis. As his sense of Self developed, he became able to feel he belonged in the world as an important part of creation, and strong enough to understand and forgive his parents who were hurt as children too.

How You Can Avoid the Seven Deadly Spirit Traps

In a sense, all disturbed people have sold their soul to the devil. Having lost their sense of worth, integrity, and love, they are driven by their anxiety to lie to themselves and present a false self to the world. Their inner tension and hostility have replaced their natural good feelings. This is the hell of spiritual alienation. The devil emerges when our reason is perverted by feelings of fear and hostility; when we become inwardly self-destructive and outwardly immoral. The myth of Lucifer symbolizes this fall. The power of light and reason turn against God (our wholeness and goodness) to become the Prince of Darkness.

1. Pride: The Cardinal Sin

The seven deadly sins of religious psychology are identical with clinical symptoms of depth psychology and psychiatry. The cardinal sin, false pride, is the restless state of egocentricity. Fear and hostility motivate the personality and alienate one from the loving and harmonious Self, from self-worth and inner freedom. Since the Self (see the Personality Chart) is the basis of our emotional and spiritual health and sanity, all the other sins or symptoms stem from the loss of this healthy state.

The person who is filled with conceit is always lacking in genuine self-worth. Egotism is a painful state of separation from reality in which driven people desperately try to show themselves and the world that they are "somebody." Whatever outer success may appear in the clever facade, inner feelings of anxiety and guilt remain.

Anxiety or chronic fear stems from the sense of being

separated from God or the Life Force. This alienation from the Source—the sustaining power of the cosmos—is always accompanied by physical rigidity and tension. "Stiff-necked pride" is also a physical attitude that splits the mind from the body and damages the unity of the person (with himself or herself and with the Creator). This tension blocks energy and causes negative emotions, like a dammed-up stream that stagnates or finally breaks out and runs wild. In very disturbed people, this is the manic-depressive syndrome. In this condition, the mind knows no peace and is endlessly driven to maintain pretenses and to worry incessantly that they might be seen through.

Guilt feelings also accompany false pride, when the inner and outer person are disparate. This sense of wrongness cannot be shaken, for deep inside there remains an awareness that one is out of tune with life. Unfortunate attempts have been made to avoid spiritual dis-ease and guilt through drugs, alcohol, pseudosexuality, material possessions, power, prejudice, masochism, violence, and superficial religiosity—involving the four dimensions of the human being. But Saint Augustine's affirmation remains true: "Our hearts cannot rest until they rest in Thee." (See Chart: The Happy State.)

In the infant, there is no boundary between the self and the outside world. Gradually we learn to distinguish between them, and we develop an ego, a sense of a separate self. As we mature, it is necessary to slough off that ego (that sense of separation) in the same way that a snake drops its old skin. Then instead of being self-conscious and trapped in our petty egos, we become conscious of Self as an infinitesimal but nonetheless important part of the Life Force.

Only when we give up our pride can we relax our guard and become capable of drawing a free breath. The aspect of breathing—though left out of conventional psychoanalysis—

is an important part of Syntonic therapy. Breath is life, and
by freeing the tensions that block deep breathing, one can
begin to experience the life that flows through and unifies our
body, mind, and spirit. The Hindu sages spoke of *Atman*—
this inner energy—as being One with Brahman, the infinite
Life Force. Going beyond one's ego, discovering that state of
being that I call the real Self, has been called enlightenment,
maturity, Christ consciousness, salvation—all descriptive of
the process of outgrowing false pride and discovering Self-
esteem. And Self-esteem is the cornerstone of the whole personality; physical health, emotional well-being, peace of
mind, and spiritual joyfulness. These four human dimensions
are interrelated. Depending on whether they are negative or
positive, one becomes more isolated by tension, fear, and
doubt; (the fight or flight system) or grows toward greater
well-being and fulfillment (the parasympathetic state). "The
fruits of the Spirit are love, joy and peace." (Galatians 5:22) I
believe all therapies and all religions are based on this polar-
ity of the autonomic nervous system. (See Personality Chart.)

Atheists and agnostics are out of touch with the Life
Force and hold negative beliefs which create self-fulfilling
prophecies of negative experiences. They approach reality
from a negative state of mind, unaware that "out of the heart
are the issues of life." The more you love the Creative Power
that sustains the cosmos and the awesome syntony of our
trillions of cells, the more Divine Power flows through your
being, dissolving fear and deadness and egotism and bringing serenity, joy, and a sense of your own divinity.

Many "believers," however, misuse their religion as a tool
of the ego, to make themselves superior and to dominate
those of other faiths. Truly, "the Devil can quote Scripture
to his own purposes." A recent example of this attitude was
a Baptist leader who proclaimed that "God Almighty does

not hear the prayer of a Jew." The irony of this pettiness was pointed out by another Baptist, who suggested that his colleague "pause long enough to realize that Jesus was a Jew, a loyal and faithful Jew. Does that mean that God would not hear Him?" It is difficult to underestimate the mayhem caused by "religious" fanatics driven by pride and its unholy trinity of fear, hatred, and greed.

In contrast, true religion teaches the wholeness and holiness of creation. In the words of a living Indian guru, Sai Baba, "Wherever Truth, Peace and Love are emphasized — in whatever religion or language — by whichever teacher, there we have the *eternal religion.*"[1]

Pride is based on the illusion of separateness and on creatures oblivious to their Creator: In Shakespeare's words, "All is vanity and vexation of spirit." Energy that is short-circuited by tension and fear becomes destructive within and without. Clinically this is described as masochism or sadism. In electricity, negative and positive poles must be brought together to produce light. The union of human consciousness and the Cosmic Energy results in enthusiasm, joy, vitality, pleasure, and enlightenment.

A Lady of Desperation

False pride or egotism, which stems from a lack of awareness of one's real Self and connection with God, is a major part of every variety of emotional and mental disorder.

A very bright, attractive, and cultured young women sought my help recently. She had read a book of mine and told me on the phone that she had to see me immediately, for

---

[1] *Sathya Sai speaks,* New Jack Printing Works, Bombay, India, 1979.

she was convinced that I would have the answer to her problems. I assured her that I would do my best to help her help herself. Sensing her desperation, I juggled my schedule so that I could see her the same day.

She was a very distraught woman, and she told me even before sitting down that she had no problems, had had a happy childhood, but she just "had" to get a particular man she knew to marry her. After being seated, she raced through the story of their relationship. He was bright, successful, cultured, and all she ever wanted. With other men she had always been bored, but with him, passion and excitement knew no bounds.

When I asked if there were anything wrong with him or their relationship, she began to cry. He was a compulsive worker who was involved in business over twelve hours a day; he would lie to her and spend nights with other women; and worst of all, his moods would turn hot and cold. At times he was unable to be away from her; while at other times he insisted that it was all over and she should find someone worthy of her.

I played back her description of this very disturbed man—his tension, unreliability, mendacity, immaturity, desperation, and lack of self-worth. I asked her what she would advise a woman friend who might wish to marry such a man, and she said, "Get rid of him." This was her rational Self speaking. She herself was very immature and insecure beneath a facade of a chic, sophisticated woman of the world. Birds of a feather do seem to flock together! The egoistic child part of her, her unconscious, had to marry this man. She was anxious, bored, and deadened, and to feel alive she needed his psychological whippings.

The ultimate concern of her life was to marry a man she neither trusted nor respected. The false god whom she wor-

shipped (one thinks of the biblical warning against wor-
shipping "graven images") was an idealized image of the
man she intellectually knew to be disturbed and helpless,
despite financial conquests. Lacking a sense of Self and self-
worth, she was driven by false pride to weep and denigrate
herself when he rejected her. I pointed out that a self-
respecting woman might take this bad behavior from a man
once. But if the man refused therapeutic help, she would
surely move on to a better chapter in her life. At that point,
she admitted that she was furious with him and with herself.
But she never showed her real feelings, for fear of losing
him. He in turn would feel guilty that she was such a saint,
and he was threatened by her desperate clinging.

The old theme of the desperate ego returned. "But what
can I do when I see him tonight to get him to marry me
before he goes away on a business trip?" I quoted the
Chinese saying, "Be careful what you want, you may get it."
I suggested that they were both insecure and disturbed people who needed help to grow toward emotional maturity *in
themselves* before they were ready for a commitment of marriage. In the meantime, she might start being, for once, honest with him about her anger; her saintly role was making
her tense, weak, and anxious and pushing him farther away.
At least if she lost him, she would have the beginning of self-
respect and lessen the stress she was putting on herself.

She agreed to return for therapy, and she expressed how
different this visit was from the conventional, passive psy-
chiatrist she had previously consulted. She also wanted to
convince her lover to see me as soon as possible. I explained
that I could work no miracles and that I would inform him
that he too would need help to mature emotionally, psychologically, and spiritually before marriage became a realistic
possibility.

2. Covetousness

Covetousness is the neurotic effort to relieve one's inner emptiness and anxiety by means of acquiring material possessions, which are valued above all else and accumulated at any cost. Material things are not bad in themselves, but the love of them *beyond all else* is a symptom of greed and desperation. Like the alcoholic, addict, compulsive eater, or gambler, the compulsive acquisitor sacrifices everything in his or her obsession. No doubt Jesus had this attitude in mind when he said, "It is easier for a camel to pass through the eye of a needle than a rich man to enter the Kingdom of Heaven." (Mark 10:25)

Wes, the Incurable Millionaire

Wes was an arrogant multimillionaire on the outside but was a tortured soul within. His inner child felt empty and worthless due to a lonely childhood in a mansion without affection from either parent. Feeling unlovable, Wes was incapable of experiencing good feelings about himself or anyone else. Flaunting his money to "prove" his worth as a person alienated people, which in turn drove him to even greater attempts to impress with his wealth.

I felt a deep compassion for Wes and tried to encourage him to seek help and find a way out of the terrible vicious circle he was trapped in. However, his fear and arrogance made him unreachable. There is a Russian proverb: "Only the grave can cure the hunchback."

Prudishness undermines the love life of humans, and pornography is the opposite side of the coin. Wes was too cold and fearful to love, and used his money to buy sex. Without a happy love life and the joy and fulfillment that genuine sexuality brings, material possessions become his ultimate concern—the false god—of those who cannot love. But like all false religions, it yields worry, anxiety, and illness rather than gratitude and happiness. William James spoke of it as "the bitch goddess success."

Whether one covets money, fame, power, a title, one's own child, one's lover or mate as an end in itself rather than as a gift to be valued and respected, the result is always damaging.

Tim, the Attorney who Coveted Little Boys

Tim had read my book *Overcoming Homosexuality*[2] and was hopeful that my Syntonic approach to therapy might help him, as it had many other motivated men and women with this lifestyle. His experience with conventional therapy had been lengthy, expensive, and not very helpful. In his thirties, Tim's illusion of finding a stable and loving relationship with another man had faded, and his attempts to relate to women had also failed. His real sexual excitement was connected with preteenage boys. As an attorney, he realized that he was living on the edge of disaster.

Tim's family life had been miserable since infancy. His mother was anxious and explosive; his father, a passive provider. His earliest memory was a recurrent dream in which he was chased by a witch and woke up sweating, just before she caught him. As a child he was sickly and pampered by his mother, who did not want him to get hurt playing with other boys. She kept him home with her. When he came to me for help, Tim still called his mother two or three times a day to let her know that he was all right. When his parents fought, his mother would force him to take sides and decide who was right. If he sided with his father, she screamed in a hysterical fit. His only comfort had been sex play with another boy—the root of his present fixation on males, along with his aversion to females (stemming from his overpowering mother).

---

[2] Robert Kronemeyer, *Overcoming Homosexuality*, Macmillan Pub., N.Y., 1979.

Tim's mother had coveted him as an object, a possession that would give her empty life some meaning. Out of fear and guilt, he acquiesced to her obsession with him. Since all women were threatening to him as mother figures and homosexual men were frightening and usually incapable of the love and fidelity that he craved, Tim was only capable of having positive, sexual feelings with boys.

Genuine love always contains respect. Tim's mother's possessiveness was a symptom of her alienation from the Life Force and her lack of a sense of Self. Driven to make her son the center of her existence, she was unable to love him and respect his right to be, to feel, and to grow as an individual. Tim remained a frightened, spiteful child, unhappy with himself and a failure in his career, still seeking boys to play with.

Tim had to struggle with his fear, hopelessness, spite, and self-destructive rage. Through intensive Syntonic therapy, he gradually became strong enough to free himself from the inner witch who had possessed him. As he matured, he began to find his real Self, and liking himself, he was finally able to relate to and care for a woman whom he could trust and respect.

3. Lust

Lust is the compulsive need to release one's anxiety and tension through loveless sex. It is a "deadly sin" not in the sense that sex is bad, but rather because one uses another person as an object and uses sexuality as a separate part of one's wholeness. Thus lust never leads to happiness, trust, or fulfillment, but results instead in feelings of guilt and emptiness.

The most difficult lesson is to learn that first one must find comfort and happiness in oneself, in relation to God or the Life Force. Until we find inner peace and wholeness, no one else can fill our emptiness and provide security or happiness.

To put "first things first" is not easy, but to remain a child and look to someone else for happiness is more difficult and painful in the long run, for such an attitude is doomed to fail.

Mature people realize that sexuality is a *part* of life which has meaning and fulfillment physically, emotionally, mentally, and spiritually as *part* of a relationship which includes trust, honesty, and respect. Only when each person has a sense of Self can a relationship develop that is giving rather than exploitive.

Divorce statistics reveal how few people reach this level of maturity. Most marriages are based on wrong motives and are entered into by people who have not learned to be whole in themselves. Contemporary education is concerned with subject matter alone, not with growth of personality and self-awareness. "Know thyself" is the crowning goal of life, but it is only paid lip service (see Appendix IV).

Recently a religious leader made a statement in which he warned married couples against having lust for one another. I discussed this with a married couple, who thought he was saying that sex should not be enjoyed in marriage. If I understand him correctly, I believe he meant that one should respect and revere one's mate and the sexual act itself as a gift of God—not simply the means to derive selfish pleasure from an object. I agree with this point of view.

When limited as an end in itself, sex loses its meaning in so many marriages, when energies are not recharged through a spiritual connection with the Life Force or Holy Spirit.

Jon: Who Outgrew Lust and Found His Mate

A bright, handsome, and successful doctor whom I shall call Jon came to me for therapy. He complained of anxiety, depression, and irritability. His work as a surgeon began to suffer from his disturbance. Among other self-destructive habits which Jon could not overcome, he smoked excessively.

Jon had experienced relationships with hundreds of women in the course of his thirty sexually active years. He remembered several special women with whom he felt love, but in each case he had pulled back emotionally in the relationship and had provoked the woman to reject him. A frightened little boy who had never grown up was still (unconsciously) running the life of this talented and charming man.

Like all people with difficulties, Jon was physically tense, emotionally insecure, mentally worried, and spiritually empty. Mature people who have had sufficient loving and nurturing during childhood outgrow dependence on mother and father and become grounded, secure, and independent. Their only dependence rests on the Sustaining Power of the cosmos. Thus, they can relate to others with a sense of inner confidence and fullness, enjoying a relaxed body and a calm mind.

Jon was still looking for a woman (unconsciously mother) to give him love and security, but at the same time he was afraid of being dependent like a child. Thus the closer he moved toward a woman, the more he panicked and had to get away! His hit-and-run sexuality was devoid of connection with his heart, mind, and spirit. He sought sexual release to achieve relief from loneliness, but gratified lust alone could not satisfy the needs of his whole being. Pleasure becomes joy and orgasmic fulfillment only when two people deeply share with one another and merge in the Life Force itself.

Jon gradually overcame his tension, fear, and sense of alienation through Syntonic therapy, in which his sadness, fear, and rage were experienced, released and understood deeply. Gradually his blame of others gave way to his taking responsibility for his own thoughts, feelings, and behavior; and guilt and hostility melted into forgiveness. He also outgrew the atheism he affected as part of his cynical, detached attitude toward life, and he discovered the profound meaning of the rejected religion he had learned as a child. Instead of loneliness, he began to discover the richness of solitude that is available when one is connected to the Higher Power.

As Jon cultivated his inner richness ("the Kingdom of God is within you"), he relaxed into a confidence which made room for kindness toward himself and others. With much to give, he was now able to approach women in a genuinely outgoing manner, rather than feeling desperate to use them and then escape. Quite naturally, his lust turned to love. He learned to discriminate, to choose partners. He found meaning and happiness in sexual love that as a Don Juan he had never even suspected.

However disturbed a person may be, underneath there is always a healthy God-given core—a whole Self. When mind, heart, and genitals are separated by fear and tension, fulfillment is impossible. One must first become a loving, Syntonic person before becoming a lover.

One must love Being itself before one can love another person, as well as one's fellows. Dr. Erich Fromm wrote, in *The Art of Loving* "Because one does not see that love is an activity, a power of the soul, one believes that all that is necessary to find it is the right object, and that everything goes by itself afterward."

Jon had found the right object many times. But he could only lust—and lust without love is not enough to provide meaning in one's life. Love, that "power of the soul," involves one's whole being and connects us with Being itself. No wonder it is written that "God is love." Our power to love is our greatest gift from God. It is the Cosmic Energy that created us, enabling us to grow from one cell to trillions of cells, flowing through us, so that we may share in the wonder of creation.

When he went deeply within to find his Self and removed the debris of tensions and distortions that had impeded his way, Jon discovered the capacity to trust and love that he had lost in infancy. The French scientist Dr. Frederick LeBoyer points out in *Birth Without Violence* that the cold, mechanical birthing that humans inflict on their young sets the stage for the lovelessness (the fight or flight state) that plagues the human race. Jon's intensive syntonic therapy enabled him to free his heart, mind, and body from his earliest fears and open the natural pathways of love (the parasympathetic state). No longer driven by lust to empty, desperate sex, he discovered that making love is the fruit of the spirit of loving.

4. Hostility

The disturbed person whose energy is blocked by fear seesaws between passivity and aggression. In a passive state and lacking self-respect, one can easily be exploited. In contrast, the healthy person has a sense of Self and inner well-being, is able to enjoy a natural flow of energy, and is positively self-assertive, demonstrating respect for others and for himself or herself. Unlike the fearful person who clings to a relationship that is destructive, the mature individual is secure enough to *leave* a situation in which the other person is incapable of respect, though he or she may glibly speak of love.

Many relationships are cemented together by mutual and partly unconscious hostility. Each partner dreads being alone and needs an outlet for his or her negativity. This release of negative feelings prevents such people from facing their unbearable depression and alienation from reality. The degree of destructiveness is in proportion to the frustration of the need for physical, emotional, mental, and spiritual satisfaction. In the spiritual dimension, the hostile person experiences being alone as loneliness; the healthy person, in contact with the Life Force, enjoys solitude as an experience of re-creation.

In *Escape from Freedom,* Dr. Fromm describes this deadly state of neurotic aggression:[3] "The more the drive toward life is thwarted, the stronger is the drive toward destruction; the more life is realized the less is the strength of destructiveness. Destructiveness is the outcome of un-lived life."

There is a vast array of clinical evidence for the deadly effects of hostility, destructive anger, and aggression on human life. This dis-ease results in psychosomatic illnesses ranging from headaches, backaches, fatigue, and indigestion to ulcers and heart attacks. There is also research to substantiate that arthritis and cancer may be related to frustration and blocked or disturbed aggressiveness.

In *Type A Behavior and Your Heart,* the cardiologists Drs. Roseman and Friedman suggest that this kind of person—constantly hurried, overcompetitive, worried, who is hostile in every traffic jam and bristles when having to wait on line—is prone to suffer a heart attack. Being tense, egoistic, and inclined toward rage is indeed a deadly sin. From a wholistic point of view, it can be seen as a behavior disorder that can also be helped by eliminating stress-producing substances from one's diet: sugar, caffeine, drugs, junk foods, fatty meats, and excessive alcohol. Breathing exercises and self-relaxing techniques, hypnosis, meditation, and the elimination of neurotic and obsessive thinking also help.

I remember skiing in the Alps some years ago with a group of new acquaintances, one of whom was a robust man in his forties who was driven to make more runs down the mountain than anyone else. He gulped his lunch and was off again while the rest of us basked in the winter sun,

---

[3] Healthy aggression means to move forward in the world in a positive manner; it might more properly be called assertiveness.

rested after lunch and enjoyed warm fellowship and the fabulous views of distant peaks. I wondered how long he would last in his desperate attempt to fight the world and build his ego. I later learned that he had died of a heart attack the following year.

Jan: Who Grew From Hostility to Assertiveness

Jan was a talented dancer who came for therapy because of her anxiety, agitation, and depression. Her husband was afraid to come for help himself, though he suffered from similar symptoms, along with asthma attacks and drinking binges. He said he loved her but showed no consideration for her feelings and needs. Sexually he was only concerned with his own desires, and he lacked any tenderness and empathy in relation to his wife. He insisted on going out with his friends, but he became insanely jealous if Jan did anything or saw anyone without him.

Tension mounted inside Jan until she exploded. Usually the fights between Jan and her husband were verbal, but occasionally violence on the part of her husband would occur, leaving Jan bruised and humiliated. Too afraid to even consider leaving the house or calling the police, she would suffer quietly until the next outburst.

In therapy Jan began to see that she was acting out her childhood pattern of not feeling loved by her parents, and then provoking them to punish her. As she released the tension and pain stored up since childhood, she began to understand that her hostile behavior was masochistic and counterproductive. She used syntonic techniques to feel her power and anger rather than merely verbalize it. She learned to let her husband know that she was hurt by his attitudes, rather than attacking him for them and feeding into his hostilities. Experiencing herself as a whole person and finding strength through spiritual awareness,

Jan lost the trait of being a desperate child needing love from someone unable to give it. She began to understand and feel compassion for her disturbed and immature husband.

As part of her therapy, Jan used emotional release techniques, after which she played a tape which I made to help her redirect herself and take responsibility for her feelings and thoughts. She grew into a more secure and assertive woman. I do not know what happened with her marriage, but I do have faith that as she becomes stronger she will only stay in this marriage if her husband is willing to get help for himself. If he cannot or will not make real changes, Jan will be able to be alone and enjoy solitude, because she is finding her Self and a spiritual awareness of the Life Force. At some point I believe she will find someone with self-esteem who is worthy of her; someone at her level of maturity.

5. Gluttony

The actuarial tables of insurance companies leave no doubt about the deadliness of compulsive overeating. The strain of carrying extra weight adds further stress to an organism already disturbed by tension and anxiety. Gluttony is a symptom of emotionally disturbed persons who have lost their spiritual connection with the Life Force. Desperately they try to fill their inner emptiness and push down their fear, sadness, and rage with food. Essentially, they are driven by the same demons as gluttons for drugs, cigarettes, and alcohol. The fatter they get, the more they hate themselves, and the more they hate the more they eat.

Gluttons are not aware of how much they eat. Often they eat normal amounts during the day, in public, but during the night the desperate inner child indulges in voracious and uncontrolled eating. Although there may be glandular imbalances and genetic or inherited factors in gluttonous behavior, there are always psychological and emotional factors stemming from a disturbed infancy and an unhappy childhood. Food becomes a substitute for (mother) love and a way of deadening emotional pain and stress. The distressed inner child in the gluttonous adult seeks food as a pacifier, whereas other disturbed individuals are driven to drugs, alcohol, smoking, or compulsive work or sex.

Jay: Whose Weak Inner Child Grew to Manhood

Jay had been a college athlete weighing 180 pounds, which for his height and structure was a normal weight. After graduation, the pressures of being out in the world and having to prove himself and be self-supporting inflamed the deep fears and self-doubts that he had been keeping under control. Additionally, he was no longer athletically active, and he used food to bury his fears and his deep ambivalence toward women. Within two years, he had blown up to 265 pounds.

Jay had always suffered from lack of self-worth and a sense of impending disaster. Such reactions were appropriate and understandable since Jay's mother was cold and critical, and his father was a weak and frightened man who abused alcohol and fluctuated between hostile fighting with his wife and periodic bouts of depression, guilt, and withdrawal. Food was the one sign that his parents cared and the only positive, pleasurable experience that Jay could count on. Little wonder that he turned to food in a desperate attempt to relieve his inner emotional pain and panic. The vicious circle in which he was caught finally drove him to seek therapeutic help.

Fortunately he found Syntonic therapy, which encouraged him to give vent to his fear, sadness, and rage rather than merely discussing and analyzing his emotions. Catharsis enabled him gradually to release his pent up emotions and understand their causes. I encouraged Jay to act out in therapy his negative feelings toward members of his family. As long as there is buried hatred, one remains physically tense and mentally confused, since the body and the mind are one.

Jay learned to use his rage as a positive force, by pounding cushions, kicking and stamping. He overcame his fears, tensions, negative images, and thoughts that had kept him short-circuiting his energies and constantly defeating himself. As he resolved the conflicts and behavior patterns that undermined his self-esteem and kept him tangled in the inner child, he became more assertive, positive, and reasonable in solving his problems. When securely grounded on his own two feet and aware of the joy of being in touch with the Life Force, his gluttony and overweight were discarded. No longer afraid of life, his protective armor of tension and fat were no longer necessary and melted away!

6. Envy

Envy is the sign of a blown-up ego and the lack of an inner sense of Self. A hostile preoccupation with the good fortune of others (real or imagined) stems from a lack of pleasure and joy in living. Often the envious are materially successful but, being emotionally and spiritually bankrupt, they are never grateful for what they have and never satisfied no matter how much they accumulate. Their inner chronic dissatisfaction drives them with deadly precision to the eventual destruction of everything they possess.

As finite humans, the more separated we become from the Creative Power in which we live, the more prone we are to envy those who enjoy their existence. Scripture warns of the fate of those who lack spiritual peace and well-being: "To those who have, it shall be added unto them; to those who have not it shall be taken away, even that which they have." (Matthew 25:29) The philosopher La Rochefoucauld observed, "We get secret pleasure from the misfortune of our friends." I reject the total cynicism of this blanket statement. However, when we are out of tune with the universe and disturbed, it is true that our energies cannot flow with genuine compassion. Lacking wholeness of mind and body, we say words without feeling them in our hearts.

Zen Flesh, Zen Bones by Paul Reps contains a story called "The Voice of Happiness." A sage called Bankei found the serenity and joy that comes with wholeness and enlightenment. After Bankei's death, a blind man who lived nearby told a friend that he judged the character of others by the sound of their voices. Ordinarily, the man said, when someone congratulates another upon his happiness or success, I also hear a tone of envy. And when condolence is expressed for the misfortune of another, he continued, the one condoling often sounds glad there is something left to gain in his own world. In all my experience, however, Bankei's voice was always sincere. Whenever he expressed happiness, I heard nothing but happiness, and whenever he expressed sorrow, sorrow was all I heard."

Enid, Whose Rage to Live Overcame Her Bulimia and Envy

A young woman, whom I shall call Enid, came for therapy. She was suffering from crippling fear and guilt that resulted in her tending to withdraw periodically from reality and to hide in her apartment. She was bright and attractive but constantly envious of anyone who appeared to be smarter than she. She was also obsessed with the idea that the thinner she was, the more attractive she was. When she was driven by her fear and tension to eat compulsively, she learned to vomit afterward. The vomiting not only kept her from getting overweight, but it also served as a release of tension. In therapy, Enid discovered that when she became anxious about others being smarter and brighter than she, her throat and neck would become so tight that she felt on the edge of insanity and that her mind was splitting from her body.

Enid's father was a physician and had taken her to orthomolecular psychiatry and psychoanalysis for several years. At times he had her hospitalized in an attempt to help her change her self-destructive behavior. Only when she was able to experience her deeply buried (unconscious) negative emotions and dissolve her crippling bodily tensions was Enid able to begin to use her energies in a rational way. The story of her struggle would take a book in itself. Suffice it to say that through the warm support and the dynamic techniques of Syntonic therapy, Enid began to move out toward the world. By pounding cushions, kicking and yelling, and expressing her rage to live she became stronger and freer, and developed genuine insight.

Instead of living as a desperate infant—eating and vomiting and curling up into herself—Enid began to study again and finished college, and then won a scholarship to graduate school. Whenever she became envious of someone whom she felt was brighter, however, she panicked and ran home to act out the eating-vomiting ritual. There was a part of her that she could not control, she explained, and this part seemed to take over beyond her control. After each episode she was stricken with remorse and vowed never to repeat this behavior again; finally she was able to maintain her Self and her own self-esteem.

Another part of the web of her neurosis involved her guilt about sexuality. Her family and upbringing had been strictly Catholic, puritanical, and antisexual. She had been taught that the punishment of extramarital sex was eternal hellfire. As a child she had a nightmare in which Jesus appeared to accuse her of being worse than Satan. (This is reminiscent of a theme in

James Joyce's *Portrait of the Artist as a Young Man*. Joyce portrayed the pitiless damage to the psyche by pseudo-religious rejection of the body. In any true religion, however, the body is accepted and respected as the wonderful creation it is, "the temple of the Spirit.")

Enid has developed a relationship with a man but has yet to overcome her fear of giving herself in sexual love. The fear of losing her ego and her tendency to be centered in her head still keeps her from surrendering to love in true sexual fulfillment. Unable to relax completely, Enid still worries about other students in a competitive way. She no longer runs home to release her tension and sense of depersonalization by eating and vomiting. She has learned to challenge these thoughts and to use tension release techniques as an alternative to infantile compulsion. A cassette tape used in conjunction with therapy aids in helping her maintain her equilibrium, her sense of Self, despite outer stresses of her life.

Enid is in the last phase of getting well. As she relaxes further and becomes emotionally centered, assertive, and mentally clear, she is also growing in spiritual contact with the Life Force and enjoying good feelings. Her old distorted concept of a destructive god is being replaced by a living experience of the positive Creative Power of the universe. When she deepens her capacity to unify her sexuality with the power of love, her envy will completely disappear like mist before a rising sun.

7. Sloth

Sloth is a state of inactivity and depression in which the natural vitality of a person is blocked by fear and tension. Some people act out their fear by attacking others; others cling to and covet others as objects to be possessed; the depressive person withdraws and resigns from the struggle of living.

The roots of this condition go back to the deprivation of love, warmth, and closeness in the earliest years of life. This undermines the natural well-being of the human organism and creates a reservoir of negative emotions: fear, chronic sadness, and anger. The expression of these feelings in childhood is usually punished in some way by inadequate parents devoid of insight and maturity. (This process is described in the Personality Chart.) The stronger children rebel and become hostile, the weaker cling and submit, and the weakest tend to give up and resign.

The latter group have lost their potential for faith, hope, and love by choosing inaction as the safest course. If one withdraws and does nothing, at least one finds safety in not behaving in a wrong way. "Selling one's soul to the devil" — giving up one's self-esteem and aliveness for survival — is always accompanied by painful feelings of guilt and unhappiness. Underlying feelings of rage are turned against oneself in self-denial, against others in spiteful passivity, and against life itself in cynicism and despair. This state of spiritual illness and separation from the Life Force is devastating to human dignity, and one is caught in the deepest circles of hell.

Dan, Who Overcame Homosexuality and Became Heterosexual

Dan, a sensitive young man in his late twenties, looked like a thin, shy child. His whole being seemed to express the attitude, "excuse me for existing." His voice was so constricted that it was almost inaudible; his eyes were averted and downcast; his fingers constantly played with each other to remind him that they were really there; his feet were often placed one on top of the other, as if to avoid contact with the floor and any affirmation of his right to be; his back and shoulders hunched over like the protective armor of a turtle. Fear is usually hidden beneath attitudes of belligerence, detachment, forced gaiety, spitefulness, hyperactivity, contempt, or bravado. Dan's own fear was raw and open; he reacted like an abandoned fawn in a cold and hostile world.

Dan never knew his real father. His mother doted on him during his formative years, clinging to him for warmth and security, using him to give meaning to her existence. A frightened child herself, she had no love to give. In desperation, she married a brutal man who hated Dan as a rival and a "mother's boy," and who occasionally beat his wife and ridiculed Dan and made him a whipping boy. Dan's spirit was undermined and crushed, and he became the scapegoat of the neighborhood bullies.

Although many people experience periods of lack of self-confidence and withdrawal, for Dan inactivity was his way of life. The safest thing to do was stay in his room and do nothing. During Dan's teens, when his stepfather was sent to prison, he felt a surge of hope. But his mother accepted the man back upon his release from jail. This was the final straw for Dan. Such a betrayal by his mother who professed "love" for him was unacceptable. He withdrew again into inactivity, torn by a smoldering rage and nagging hopelessness. His fears and feelings of inadequacy contributed to a confused sexual identity, and his occasional desperate homosexual encounters left him with painful feelings of guilt and loneliness. Attempts at conventional psychotherapy failed, for his words had little connection with his buried feelings and his rigid body. He wanted to be heterosexual but that seemed beyond reach.

Finally, Dan encountered and began to respond to Syntonic therapy. I urged him to breathe deeply and express himself through any sounds or movements that wanted to come forth, slowly reconnecting him with his buried emotions. Crying released some fear and tension. Like all people caught in fear and tension, split between mind and body, Dan had been unable to draw a free breath. For the first time he started to really breathe.

I taught him release exercises to unfreeze the energy locked in his tense musculature. Kicking out while lying on his back and pounding with his fists to unlock tension and unleash feelings in his legs and back, arms and shoulders, Dan started to come alive. Using fantasy, I encouraged him to connect these movements (and the rage to live that came into awareness) with those parts of his mother and stepfather that he hated. As he began to fight back against the dream characters, bullies, witches, and a crazy murderer who had lurked inside him, his debilitating nightmares gradually changed.

I persuaded Dan to eliminate junk foods, sugar, soda, coffee, and nicotine from his diet, for these substances only added to his anxiety by triggering his adrenals, disturbing his blood sugar balance, and depleting his vitamin supply. Whole natural foods and vitamin and mineral supplements gave him added energy to work with in the struggle for self-liberation!

Gradually Dan resynthesized his thoughts, feelings, and movements and began to regain the self-respect that comes from a feeling of wholeness. The Syntonic program was working. As his energy began to flow, he began to work more with himself at home between sessions, when old attitudes began to creep back. Afterward Dan used the cassette tape I made to help him redirect and strengthen the healthy Self.[4] However deeply buried, this healthy Self can be discovered as in the myth of the Holy Grail.

As he learned to center himself (a technique I describe in Section II), Dan began to feel his feet on the ground. He became less self-conscious as he became more conscious of his Self. He moved out to his own apartment and looked for a job so he could support himself.

---

[4] Work at home with therapeutic techniques is an excellent way for a person to outgrow dependence on the therapist and learn to help himself or herself.

The best cure for depression is expression, and the best cure for passivity is activity. As Dan's energy began to flow his posture improved, and he was able to look me in the eye. He challenged his fear of participation in a therapy group and began to speak out from his heart in a clear voice. At the same time his natural sexuality was released and he resolved his confusion over sexual identity. He no longer felt compelled to seek release with prostitutes or experiment with homosexual encounters. Now, for the first time he had an actual sexual feeling flowing through his body when he was close to a woman he liked. His comment was honest: "It scared me; it just happened. But it felt good; I'll just have to get used to good feelings."

All of the above symptoms or "deadly sins" are accompanied by a lack of joyful feeling, grace, and genuine self-love. When guilt is repressed, the last bastion against the demonic distortions in humans is overrun, resulting in psychopathic behavior. In contrast, the healthy manifestation of human dignity and spirituality has been described by Marcus Aurelius: "The good man acts the same, whether there are laws or not." And in the same vein, Saint Augustine stated, "Love God and do as you please." How sweet it is to be free!

True and False Religions

Lacking authentic spirituality that comes with the nurturing of one's capacity to trust and to love, modern humans, as Jung wrote, find themselves "in search of [their] soul." The search for the meaning of human existence is seen in the recent revival of interest in religion, demonology, the occult, astrology, consciousness raising, meditation, yoga, Eastern philosophy, and humanistic psychology. Once lost, however, the natural syntony and spirituality of the Self are difficult to regain.

Love is the binding power that unifies humans with themselves, their fellow creatures, and the universe. But the foundation of love is more often than not damaged in the early years of life. With each generation of damaged children, religion has become more socialized into suppressive practices (like those of education and law), attempting to force morality on twisted, antisocial human beings through fear and guilt. Despite knowledge of humankind's emotional and sexual nature, miseducation and false religion continue to undermine spirituality—humankind's natural contact with the Creative Energy of the universe.

False religion has created a false god, a cosmic projection of the puritanical parents who invented it. This false god, an omnipresent Peeping Tom which is the counterpart of the neurotic (piecemeal) self, is turned against the whole (holy) Self. This false god is antilife, antisexuality, and antilove. Until we can cast out our fear through the power of love, its negative power viscerally remains from childhood conditioning. Forced to "look upon" ourselves and to control the negative impulses that have been created in us, we have lost our birthright of spontaneity, inner freedom, and *joie de vivre.*

Rollo May defined puritanism as consisting of three elements: "a state of alienation from the body . . . the separation of emotion from reason . . . and the use of the body as a machine."[5] These symptoms are the result when one's emotional core is turned from a natural, loving state of being into a fear-hate orientation. (Again, the two sides of the autonomic nervous system.) Educated to hate the

---

[5] Rollo May, *Love and Will*, W. W. Norton & Co., Inc., New York, 1969.

sexual, emotional, and vital parts of our being, we hate others and life itself (despite our pretenses to the contrary). Hate, division, and destructiveness, though practiced by many religions, are the antithesis of spirituality.

A fourth element in puritanism, then, is spiritual alienation, that loss of intimacy with the Life Force, the cosmic flow, the ground of being, Allah, the Tao, Brahman, the Infinite, or whatever name one chooses. Spirituality, parental love, charity (agape) and sexual communion (eros) are expressions of the same energy. Without experiencing true sexual surrender, the *mysterium tremendum,* we are caught in our separateness, our heads, our egos. We come from two sex cells. The electrical creation we call the body is "the temple of the Spirit." The contemporary Indian guru Rajneesh writes, "right now you are a sex unit. And unless this unit is understood deeply, you cannot become spiritual. . . . Sexuality and spirituality are two ends of one energy."

Albert Schweitzer, philosopher, musician, physician, and missionary, described religion as "reverence for life." Whoever rejects, condemns, misuses the human body— one's own or someone else's—is antireligious. Often this is done in families, churches, and schools that claim to be "religious" but ironically spread the disease of sexual guilt.

Just as the body is "the temple of the Spirit," the world is the body of God. And as we pollute or waste it, or use its power for greed or war, we are pretentious and antireligious.

There are thousands of creeds, rituals, religions, and theologies. Some are petty and limited in vision; others are great and enobling. But all are derived from our longing for reunion with the Cosmic Energy of the universe. And all are like grains of sand on the beach, before the infinite ocean of Truth.

Examine your religion, your "ultimate concern" as my friend Paul Tillich would say, and see whether you are using it as a path to the top of the mountain, from which you can respect the other religions, or as a narrow alley that keeps you trapped in your arrogant little ego. Sai Baba has said, "Wherever Truth, peace and love are emphasized—in whatever religion or language—by whichever teacher, there we have the eternal religion."

The Concept of Sin

Sin is a valid label for a sick or distorted attitude. False pride is based on the illusion that one is self-created and self-sustaining, rather than the realization that every moment of life—and all existence—are given. In the former state, one is head centered (preoccupied with "me"), a prisoner of one's ego, and a victim of the endless compulsive thinking that knows no rest.

This state of spiritual alienation is always accompanied by physical tension and negative emotions. Centered in one's head, one is unbalanced and topheavy. It is rightly said that "pride goeth before the fall." In this state, the four dimensions of dis-ease and unhappiness are always present. Separated from our inner wholeness, from Oneness with the Creative Power, we are futilely driven to relieve our tension and get trapped in other "deadly sins," like gluttony, lust, greed, envy and hatred.

In contrast, the healthy state is one in which we are connected with the Life Force. Wholeness, holiness, and integration have meaning in all dimensions of human life. We talk about a whole person, an integrated personality, and someone who is "together" (that is, in tune with one's spirit or energy flow). The word *religion* means "to bind together."

Yet distorted pseudo-religions split the mind from the body. We often forget that Jesus railed most against those who "cried Lord, Lord" and failed to "do the will of the Father."

God, then, is Creative Energy in which we live and move and have our being. The word *yoga* means union, and hatha yoga exercises are ways of learning to relax our bodies and open our breathing so that the Life Force can flow. I know from studying philosophy and comparative religion for years, and looking for "the answer," that I was looking in the wrong place (outside myself) with the wrong equipment (mind alone). Only after working with therapists to dissolve my fears, guilts, and tensions, and practicing yoga, healthy nutrition, and mediation, did I begin to discover a state of inner peace in which I could glimpse the meaning of Saint Augustine's dictum: "Our hearts cannot rest until they rest in Thee." Note the emphasis on the heart, the emotional facet. Only when the heart is free of chronic fear and hate can the body relax and the mind be serene. Thus only the "pure in heart" can know God and are able to experience Oneness.

Western civilization has largely only paid lip service to this wisdom and to the wisdom of the Delphic oracle, to "know thyself." We thought that by conquering nature we could bring happiness to the world. Our education has focused on knowledge alone, without the understanding that comes from the heart, the spirit, and the body. A. S. Neill warned us of this in his book *Hearts Not Heads in the Schools*, about Summerhill School in England.

The twentieth century is replete with unspeakable cruelties brought about by scientific ingenuity in the service of fear, greed, hatred, and arrogance. Affluent citizens of this affluent society are rarely happy—crime, neurosis, divorce, illness, loneliness, depression, and addiction plague the rich as well as the poor. How could it be otherwise?

We have neglected to teach our youth to be self-aware, to meditate, strengthen their physical health through sound nutrition, and to take responsibility for their own inner peace, sexuality and happiness. We need experiential groups at all stages of education, and a Department of Personal Growth in every school and college, to focus on emotional growth, compassion, and self-knowleldge. To "Know Thyself" should be the *primary* goal of education; to develop caring and positive human beings who will be good parents, neighbors and citizens!

Raised in the Protestant tradition, I learned the two great commandments: "First love the Lord thy God with all thy heart, soul and mind; and the second is like unto it; love thy neighbor as thyself." But I had been conditioned as a child to think of God as able to watch me at all times, especially after Mother had me put my hands together in prayer outside the bed covers before sleeping. When I went to college, my study of evolution and astronomy led me to agnosticism. It was impossible to love a God about whose existence I was so uncertain. Nor could I truly love myself or others since deep fears, guilt, and tension blocked the free flow of energy. Now I know one must be "pure in heart," free of fear and hate to truly know God. One must experience this wholesome state of being to understand the words, "God is love."

The Four Steps to Syntonic Wholeness

Several years ago, I discovered a practical method of achieving the state of balance and harmony in the Japanese system called Aikido. In Japanese, *ai* means "harmony," *ki* means the "Life Energy," and do means the "way": "the way of harmony with the Life Energy." The master who taught and inspired me is Koichi Tohei.

Aikido teaches that the mind and the body are one. We lose this harmony and Oneness in the course of our development and head-centered education. To the extent that the mind separates from the body, we are mentally and emotionally sick, (a split personality). Lacking the inner harmony that is necessary to feel Oneness with the universe, we feel empty, disturbed, and estranged. As we have seen, this egoistic state of alienation leads to other deadly patterns of behavior.

In Aikido I was amazed to discover that their four rules parallel the four interrelated dimensions of the human personality which I developed in Syntonic therapy. The motto of Aikido as expressed by Master Tohei is as follows: "Let us have a universal spirit that loves and protects all creation and helps all things grow and develop. To unify mind and body and become one with the universe is the ultimate purpose of my study." In a simple and beautiful way, does this motto not embody the essense of the two Judeo-Christian commandments, "love God and thy neighbor as thyself"? These are the four rules of Aikido:

1. *Keep one point.* This means constant awareness of one's center or *hara,* just below one's navel. Such awareness keeps one's mind calm and focused. "The universe is a limitless circle with a limitless radius. Condensed, this becomes the one point in the lower abdomen which is the center of the universe. Let us concentrate our mind in this one point and become one with and send our *Ki* constantly to the universe." [6]

---

[6] Koichi Tohei, *Ki Sayings,* KiNo Kenkyukai H.O., Tokyo, Japan, 1973.

2. *Relax completely.* This keeps one's body from tensions that block energy and disturb freedom of movement and prevent one from feeling connected with the universe. As Sensei Tohei says, "We are accustomed to having trouble with nervousness unnecessarily. Nervousness causes blood vessels to contract, making it difficult for impurities to leave the body and thus makes one susceptible to many diseases. Relaxation is truly an elixir of life. Let us spread the true method of relaxation, which enables us to meet each day with a spirit like that of a mild spring breeze. If we practice this, we need never get nervous and excited in our daily affairs."

3. *Keep weight underside.* This keeps one from being topheavy, mentally hyperactive, and prone to irrational thinking, and it brings a feeling of being emotionally secure and *settled down,* rather than being *up tight!* "The weight of objects is always naturally underside. Therefore the physical expression of living calmness is that the weight of every part of our body is also underside. Like the calm still surface of the water that reflects a flying bird, true living calmness is the condition of our mind that reflects all things clearly. This is man's original and natural state. (Note again: the parasympathetic state on the Personality Chart.) By understanding these principles, we can acquire true living calmness."

4. *Extend Ki.* Constantly picturing and directing one's life energy flowing outward keeps one in a giving, outgoing state of dynamic being. In loving *Ki,* the Cosmic Power or God, one becomes a loving person — spiritually whole. "Our lives are born of the *Ki* of the universe. Let us give thanks for being born

not as plants or animals but as lords of creation. We are one with the universe. There is no need to despond, no need to fear. The way we follow is the way of the universe, which no difficulty nor hardship can hinder. Let us always extend positive Ki and live our lives with a positive attitude."

Practicing these interrelated principles (if you truly have one you have them all, and if you lose one you lose them all) gradually leads to personal transformation. Happiness is the experience in all aspects of one's life of being in harmony with the Life Force. The healthy body is vital and relaxed and expresses itself with grace. The mature emotions manifest courage and love and express themselves in positive actions. The integrated mind is balanced and creative and expresses itself in constructive thinking. The free spirit is serene and joyful and expresses itself with enthusiasm. This is the goal of syntonic education and therapy; the syntonic human being.

The beauty of aikido is that one can practice the four rules at any time and in any place. Being in one's center can help clear the mind of disturbing thoughts; sitting with one's weight underneath and focusing on channeling energy outward can have a calming effect. A Zen saying cautions that one can find peace by meditating on the mountaintop, but the true test of a master is to keep one's center in the bustle of the city!

Just sitting quietly is not enough in the quest for the "truth that sets one free." True power and serenity can only be realized if one knows how to unify one's mind and body with Ultimate Reality. This is done by practicing the four basic rules that describe man's natural and healthy state of being.

At this moment, put your awareness on your center, just below your navel, and feel your weight underneath. Does your mind remain busy, or does it become quiet and serene?

Testing Your Wholeness

If you are easily pushed off balance by pressure on the chest exerted by someone else, you can immediately tell that your mind and body are not coordinated. In this case the mind, too, must be unbalanced and disturbed. Similarly, if your knee can be lifted easily by another person while you are seated crosslegged, this reveals a separated mind and body. When mind and body are one, your weight is underside and you are immovable. Try this with a friend so you can strengthen your balance and wholeness. In this state, your energy and the Infinite Energy are joined and flowing together. Sitting in "meditation" without following these principles is of no lasting value.

One can lecture endlessly about the idea of sweetness. Only when one tastes and experiences sweetness, however, can one understand it, know it, and believe it!

We live in a relative world of endless, changing phenomena. Once we find our connection with the Absolute, we are no longer deluded by the relative world. By realizing that our Self is one with the Infinite, we can avoid the anxiety that is an inevitable part of being caught in the relative world! Then when we practice the four rules of our true and undisturbed Self, we can be serenely and fully *in* the world but not *of* it!

Authentic spirituality is like the keel of a sailboat. It gives steadiness in good weather, stability when storms threaten, and when the storm strikes it saves one from being capsized.

In Greek mythology, Icarus ingeniously invented wings in

order to fly. Intoxicated by his success, he flew higher and higher, approaching too closely to the sun. His wax wings melted, and he plunged to his death in the Aegean sea.

Finite as we are, caught between heaven and earth, we can never finally capture and own that state of Oneness that can quiet our minds and fulfill our heart's desire. However, the quest to become free of one's ego and find one's Self is the greatest challenge and the deepest meaning of human existence, for only in the Self can true joy, freedom, and happiness be found.

Rabindranath Tagore, an Indian poet and philosopher and Nobel laureate who lived in the nineteenth century, described the fourfold path to self-realization in some of the most profound and beautiful words ever written. The following meditation is from a group of poems called *Gitanjali,* or song offerings, which are addressed to the Divine.[7]

Life of my life —
I shall ever keep my body free,
Knowing Thy living touch is upon my limbs.
I shall ever strive to keep all untruth out from my mind
Knowing Thou hast created the light of reason in my mind.
I shall ever drive all evil from my heart and keep my love in
    flower,
Knowing Thou hast Thy seat in the inmost shrine of my
    heart.
And it shall be my endeavor to show Thee in my actions,
Knowing it is Thy power gives me strength to act.

---

[7] Rabindranath Tagore, *Gitanjali Song Offerings,* International Pocket Library, Boston, 1912. Translated from Bengali. Introduction by William Butler Yeats.

Seven Keys to Challenging the Seven Spirit Traps

- Remember that when you are in touch with your real Self—that state in which you are aware of your center, you are relaxed with your weight underneath, and you are aware of the Life Force in and around you—you are free from these deadly and damaging attitudes known as "the seven deadly sins."

- When you do get caught in pride, greed, lust, hostility, gluttony, envy, or laziness, examine the feelings and the thoughts that create these feelings and go with these disturbed states. Write them down so you can look at them objectively.

- Use the syntonic emotional release techniques to release the tension and anxiousness that underlie these driven states and distorted attitudes.

- Mobilize positive anger to challenge the thoughts and behavior you allow to sabotage you (for instance, if you are obese and driven to eat compulsively).

- Practice being in your center. Picture the Life Force flowing through every cell of your being out toward the universe, bringing you harmony and serenity.

- Write a "case illustration" like the ones in this chapter, using yourself as the subject; then visualize yourself in a free and happy state.

- Remember that virtue is its own reward. You will have greater pleasure and joy in every aspect of your life as you gradually slough off immediate gratification, tension, tiredness, fear, worry, and egotism.

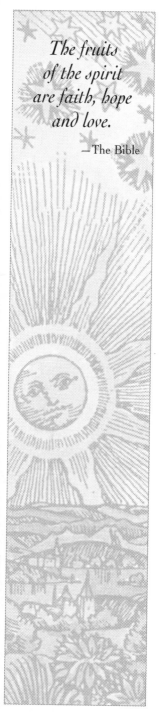

The fruits of the spirit are faith, hope and love.

—The Bible

THIRTEEN

The Syntonic View of Healthy Spirituality

Erich Fromm has written: "Man of all ages and cultures is confronted with the solution of one and the same problem: the question of how to achieve union, how to transcend over our individual life and find at-one-ment."[1] People of healthy "primitive" societies—like the Samoans, the Bantus, the Hunzas—found the answer to this question. From birth onward, they lived in harmony with

[1] Eric Fromm, *Man For Himself*, Rhinehart Pub., N.Y., 1947.

251

the laws of the universe. Through natural birth and nursing, natural nutrition, exercise, rest, relaxation, and by maintaining their innate capacity to experience pleasure, kindness, joy, and love, they remained in tune with themselves, with their fellows, and with the cosmic energy.

If "advanced" societies can learn to respect these natural laws and safeguard from birth onward the capacity for joy and love inherent in every person, (rather than the fight/flight state) man will achieve a New Age in which knowledge is combined with wisdom. If not, we will go the way of the dinosaur.

The "new" wholistic approach to humanity recognizes that we must integrate physical, emotional, mental, and spiritual knowledge for personal health and happiness. We can heal ourselves and fulfill our potential only by removing the causes of our illnesses in all four dimensions of our lives.

The Syntonic view recognizes that these four dimensions are interrelated. Thus, a therapeutic system or program for personal well-being will be most effective if it considers all dimensions of the human being. A sick body will have damaging effects on one's mind, emotions, and spirit. Irrational thinking, negative emotions, or spiritual deadness will disturb every other aspect of one's health. The famed psychic Edgar Cayce taught that "we are, physically and mentally, what we eat and what we think."[2]

The Physical Aspect of Spirituality

Throughout the ages, spiritual teachers have envisioned total Reality with a wholistic view of humankind. They saw

---

[2] Noel Langley, *Edgar Cayce on Reincarnation*, Paperback Library Inc., N.Y., 1967. Edited by Hugh Lynn Cayce.

that the physical body is a vehicle for the Life Force and that inner toxemia (the accumulation of toxins in the organs, blood, and cells) is damaging to one's aliveness of spirit.

The connection between toxemia and the modern way of living (with the refined and low fiber "diet of civilization") becomes increasingly evident. Simpler societies in which people eat less animal protein, organic vegetarian foods, and are respected for physical work are free of degenerative diseases like cancer and heart disease. These people live longer, richer lives than people in societies like ours that consume junk, refined, chemicalized foods and excess protein, lack physical exercise and self-esteem. The more toxic and obstructed the body, the greater the blockage of the Life Energy.

Religious wisdom has always recommended moderation and simplicity as virtues that are rewarded with health. The Greek philosophers celebrated "The Golden Mean." Gluttony results in sickness and premature death. The recent National Health Interview Survey conducted in Alameda County, California, revealed that the death rate of people who weighed 30 percent more than they should was two thirds higher than those of normal weight.

Let Fasting Enhance Your Spirituality

Saint Clement said, "Fasting is better than prayer." My own experience with fasting and that of many other people bears out the truth of this statement. I took two short water fasts of two and three days, respectively. I felt a bit weak and at times had a headache as the toxins began to be released from my system. Previously I had been on a "living food" diet of whole grains, raw vegetables, and fruits for several months, which had already helped me feel lighter and more vigorous. During my third fast on water and juices—this one of eight days—I experienced a feeling of energy flow, great vitality, a clearer mind, and a heightened sense of joy. I also removed the toxemia that had caused sinus trouble, arthritis, and dermatitis and was cured of these symptoms after all medical approaches had failed.

In the yoga tradition there is a saying, "In health the body is light and strong; the mind is clear and peaceful." Fasting, ideally after a transition diet of natural foods, is the quickest way to this state since it rests the body and gives it a chance to clean house. Clearing the body of toxins and tensions allows the life energy to flow freely, and one experiences intimacy with one's soul or spirit. Fasting is not for everyone, however, especially those with liver, kidney, and heart diseases. Fasts of longer than a week should be supervised by a fasting expert (a biologically oriented chiropractor or doctor). Shorter fasts should be broken with fruit for one or two days.

Many people have an automatic resistance to the idea of fasting. We are conditioned to believe that unless we eat three times a day according to the clock, we will become weak or ill. Sickness is an attempt of the body to heal itself. Instead of fasting until we are well (the instinctive wisdom of animals), we follow the mistaken voice that says, "You'd better eat to keep up your strength." After fasting I was able to do thirty push-ups, whereas on my former high-protein diet I could do only seven or eight.

If you are healthy enough to try a fast of several days, on pure water or vegetable juices, do so. Herbert Spencer, the English philosopher, wrote, "There is a principle that is a bar against all information, a proof against all argument, and which cannot fail to keep a man in everlasting ignorance. That principle is condemnation before investigation." If you listen to your body, you will know that when you are tired, sick, in pain, or emotionally upset, the natural thing to do is *not* to eat. The omission of food should ideally last until a genuine appetite and feeling of health returns. Real appetite is a sensation of watering in the mouth—*not* a tension in the gut that prompts so many people toward gluttony.

Fasting is not to be confused with starving. Our bodies store nutrients to last for several weeks or even months. This ability enabled early humans to survive in times of scarcity of food. The body uses these reserves when, in the event of sickness, food cannot be digested properly. In fasting, reestablishment of chemical balances occurs, which also has positive effects on one's mental state and spiritual aliveness. Dr. William Esser, who conducts fasting at a spa in Florida, reports that "in pernicious anemia, an increase of red cells by two or three million during the course of a three-week fast is not unusual. As accumulated waste is eliminated, a higher rate of functioning is made possible thereby in the cells and organs of the body."

A German proverb states, "The disease that cannot be cured by fasting cannot be cured by anything else." Fasting enables the remarkable powers of the human body to work and the "inner physician" to heal itself. The more healthy and toxin-free our bodies become, the more alive and in touch with the Life Force we are. This is the profound meaning of the saying, "Cleanliness is next to Godliness."

Tolstoy and his followers fasted and described their experiences as "more than a pleasure, it is the joy of the soul." The cleaner and freer our bodies become, the more we are able to be "conductors" of the cosmic electricity.

The Native Americans also understood the wisdom of fasting for self-purification and greater spiritual awareness. "Often we forget the good road in our travels. Our spirits become weak, weighted, and soiled. By fasting, sweat lodge, and self-discipline ceremonies, we cleanse and strengthen our spirit."

Jesus and Muhammed fasted for forty days and nights to experience revelations of God and the Cosmic Intelligence. The ancient Greeks knew the value of fasting for every dimension of man. Hippocrates, the "father of medicine," taught that "every man has a doctor in him; we just have to help him in his work." He warned, "to eat when you are sick is to feed your sickness." How different from the common hospital procedure today, which is to feed people who are ill with refined and processed foods.

Fasting is a way to lose weight; detoxify the body; encourage the inner miracle of healing; renew the awareness of our senses; lower cholesterol and blood pressure; feel better; relieve tension; help end dependency on such poisons as caffeine, alcohol, and nicotine; increase self-esteem; develop self-discipline; and help rejuvenate one's being. Fasting is a way to spiritual awareness. If you have health problems, seek the guidance of a wholistic doctor.

The God we discover by fasting is not the finite "God" that man has created, an imaginary being that we can placate or control. By renewing our body and spirit, we experience the Life Force that underlies all things. This Cosmic Energy created us from one cell into trillions of cells, and it sustains the beauty, majesty, order, and creativity of the inner and outer cosmos.

The Emotional Aspect of Spirituality

The First Commandment in the Bible—"Love the Lord thy God, with all thy soul, heart and mind"—(Matthew 19:18) can only be fulfilled if we respect the laws of life and maintain a healthy, vital body. For God is love, and love is the flow of cosmic energy unobstructed by bodily tensions, negative thoughts and emotions, and physical illness and toxins.

Notice again how interrelated are the four dimensions (i.e., body, emotions, mind, and spirit) of the human being. When they are in syntony we discover our soul; the joy and freedom that manifests when our Self is one with the Divine Light we call God. When we experience true physical health—not just the absence of symptoms of disease—we are simultaneously involved with positive emotions and our spirituality. Only when we are physically healthy do we feel *enthusiasm* for life; literally this word means "filled with the spirit of God." When we love the source of our being, we have an outgoing, loving attitude toward ourselves and toward others. This does not mean that we do not assert ourselves positively if through blindness or selfishness others negate our rights. But it does mean that in loving the Creator, we also feel love for creation.

The Bible contains the second commandment: "Love thy neighbor as thyself." The last two words should be stressed. To love oneself is something very few people do, for most of us are rarely lovable (i.e., in the healthy state of our true Self). When we are caught in our little egos, we are neither loving nor lovable. Only when we are in our true Self (which is shown in the center of the Personality Chart and reflects our natural state of undisturbed well-being) can we love ourself and others; then we are physically relaxed, emotionally loving, mentally clear, and spiritually in tune with the Cosmic Energy. When we lose this state, by violating the laws of life or allowing outer events or people to disturb us, we slip into the emotional unholy trinity of fear, anger, and sadness. Once again our defenses (the third circle on the chart) and the seven deadly sins take over. While thus disturbed we become caught again in our old defenses and conflicts, the "ego mind" as *A Course in Miracles* calls it, and the short circuits that block life's energy flow within. Tensions and toxins quickly build up, and inevitably old symptoms of physical, emotional, mental, or spiritual dis-ease recur.

Once again, we must return to the healthy path. The most effective way is to work with all dimensions of our being and utilize the physical, emotional, and mental techniques described in earlier chapters, followed by the spiritual exercises presented in this chapter. For this reason, it is important to make these Syntonic exercises as much a part of living as playing, working, and sleeping.

The biblical insight that "love casts out fear" was an intuition that predated by almost 2,000 years the discovery of the bipolar, autonomic nervous system. Except in emergency situations (when fear reactions are reasonable), the more we achieve inner peace and balance, the better it is for ourselves and everyone around us.

For this reason, all societies throughout history have developed ceremonies and religious institutions to help their members release tension and regain inner balance. Sometimes these institutions veer away from the true spirit of religion—always the celebration of creation and reverence for life—and degenerate into destructive social patterns of hatred and prejudice, fostering irrational guilt feelings rather than promoting social justice and inner healing.

If loving the Self is inseparable from loving the creative energy of life, it is our spiritual responsibility to become lovable persons. The more accepting we are of ourselves, the more loving we will be toward others (which means to empathize with their feelings, understand their problems, and want the best for them).

Create Love and Understanding with the Empathy Exercise

I encourage my patients to practice a loving way of relating which I call the empathy exercise. This can be done by couples, friends, student and teacher, doctor and patient, employer and employee, or parent and child—whenever people have the good will and desire to improve their relationship, diminish tension, and increase love and understanding. One person takes five minutes to try to empathize with and understand (without blame or anger) the feelings of the other person, who agrees to express his or her feelings honestly, both negative and positive. They then reverse roles for the next five minutes. This is a practical way of putting the love commandment into practice, and it is explained fully in Appendix II.

I have seen many people benefit from this procedure. Relationships often bog down because of a lack of honest communications, and negative tensions block the flow of compassion and love. The empathy exercise affords an opportunity to clear the air and release inner pressures, and it often leads to greater understanding and closeness. The empathy exercise can also be useful in relationships that are no longer viable (when it is best for people to move on to other, more appropriate relationships) because separations can often be made in the least painful and most constructive way.

Empathy Can Heal the Unhappy Family

In families, too, the use of empathy in family meetings can help lessen tension and blame, clear anxiety and anger, dissolve feelings of guilt, and strengthen mutual understanding.

The freer we are within ourselves and the more loving we feel toward others, the more we can experience the healing power and joy of life. Unhappiness and tension are inevitable when one partner dominates the other, when parents dominate children, or when children dominate parents. If you live in a tense atmosphere, empathy meetings are essential. If you find it necessary, get the help of a competent family therapist.

As a wholistic doctor, I have had many challenging experiences in treating disturbed families. Who can doubt that the family is the most important influence, for good or ill, on each human being? Unfortunately, the ill prevails. Many families are breeding grounds for physical illnesses, for the emotional plague of mass neurosis, for mental disturbances, and for spiritual stuntedness. How could it be otherwise? Most parents are totally ignorant and unprepared for the most difficult responsibility in the world—raising human lives—and blindly pass on the attitudes and errors that twisted their own growth. Ignorant of the important role of nutrition in physical and mental health, caught in their own tensions and anxieties, lacking insight into their own problems, they often pass on the sins of their parents to another hapless generation.

In all areas of health, prevention (not cure) should be the paramount concern. We must use our democratic philosophy in practice, rather than theory, in our schools to prepare the parents of tomorrow to be democratic leaders in their own families. If part of our resources and personnel were used in classes *where* the person was the subject matter—and if special teachers were trained to help students explore their thoughts, feelings, hopes, fantasies, dreams, and ways of reacting toward life and toward one another—each student would experientially learn how to be a good parent. Concern, respect, compassion, and understanding are love in action.

Such training would enable future parents to break the master-slave attitudes (sometimes the children play the master role) and change the sick family into the healthy family. In the latter, one considers the rights of others to "life, liberty, and the pursuit of happiness" (to quote the U.S. Constitution) as well as one's own.

If students' needs for help with self-understanding were met, there would be far less truancy, crime, and violent behavior in our schools. As students became more secure, they would be able to learn more effectively. To accomplish this, we need classes in which self-knowledge is the subject matter. Please see Appendix IV for a fuller discussion.

Empathy Can Lead to True Sexuality and Assertive Anger

Just as on the physical level tension and toxins that block energy create pain, so on the emotional level the toxins of negative emotions create illness and suffering. Therapeutic psychology has focused on the two major areas of life that are most often distorted—sexuality and aggression. These are the central problems in any emotional and mental disorder. They are always related to spiritual disturbances, for we become frustrated, anxious, and tense when we are out of tune with the Life Force. In this unhappy state, we are driven to a variety of compulsive behaviors.

I have defined lust as the compulsive need to release one's anxiety through loveless sex. In genuine sexual intimacy, one first feels loving within oneself and in relation to the universe. One then shares this state of well-being in sexual intimacy that is an expression of love, rather than merely a release of tension. If both partners are capable of flowing and surrender, sexuality becomes a spiritual experience in which the energy of each person merges with the other's energy and with the Life Force itself. "It's bigger than both of us" as the saying goes.

Lust may also express a compulsive need to dominate through loveless sex (even by rape) as well as by lesser degrees of exploitation by one or both members in a sexual act. To the extent that one is tense and anxious, sexuality is distorted and misused as a release for tension and anger. Since we reap what we sow, such sex is shallow and unsatisfying. To experience our real sexual potential, we must first resolve the tension and anger in ourselves, become open to the flow of life energy, clear up the problems in our relationship with empathic communication, and then enjoy lovemaking.

Destructive anger, an offshoot of fear, is an emotional "deadly sin" which destroys the state of love. The angrier we are, the more tense our bodies become. Energy is wasted in the conflict between suppression and explosion, and we increasingly lose touch with the pleasurable flow of cosmic energy. In this condition, we become spiritually bankrupt, cynical, and hopeless. In the extremes of this state, we may become a militant atheist, denying that there is any value in life whatsoever; or an agnostic, doubting the existence of the Creative Power of life. Anger is a deadly sin when it is destructive. In negative anger, we become caught in a vicious circle. In acting out negative anger, tension and anger are provoked in others.

Creative or assertive anger, however, is a positive force, directed to a positive goal. I have stressed that its most important therapeutic use is to give us the power to change our negative patterns and free ourselves from unreasonable fears and tensions. In the outer world, positive anger may be used in struggling constructively for justice, peace, educational and social improvements, and social justice. A genuine spiritual connection with the Life Force is necessary for emotional security, balance, and freedom from sexual and emotional compulsions.

Your Mind Affects Your Spirit

Religious psychology describes the way the mind can become distorted, confused, and driven to disturbed activity when, caught in the separateness of the ego, one is out of tune with the cosmic flow. In a healthy state, the mind is a source of joy, and one is free to think or not to think. Enlightenment is the realization that the mind is one's servant, and not one's master.

Irrational, distorted thought can be just as destructive to health and vitality as wrong eating, lack of rest and exercise, chronic fear, and destructive anger. To find peace and harmony, we must use our energy to challenge thoughts that keep us caught in the trap of anxiety and the fight or flight reaction. In this state of egoistic separation from our healthy Self, our minds are a never-ending source of worried compulsions that short-circuit our energy, turn us in on ourselves, and close us off from the cosmic flow. This is shown in the diagram entitled "The Egoistic State."

The unholy trinity of the mind consists of three categories of unreasonable thoughts (which we discuss next) which stem from the inner child and the negative parent parts of ourselves. Had we been loved enough in our early years and encouraged to grow as unique individuals, we would have maintained the basic feeling of self-respect and security that underlies rational thought. This is not the case in most homes and schools at this time in human evolution.

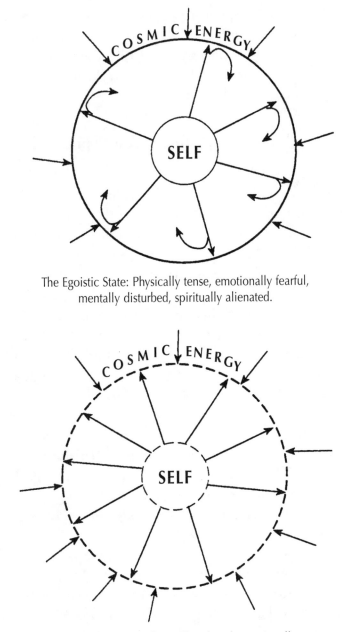

The Egoistic State: Physically tense, emotionally fearful, mentally disturbed, spiritually alienated.

The Happy State: Physically relaxed, emotionally loving, mentally serene, spiritually joyful.

Musts

Disturbed thinking often involves the word *must*. The unreasonable demands that we experienced in childhood cause exaggerated and negative self-criticism in later life. Often we tell ourselves that we *must* be perfect or else we are miserable failures. This leads to a destructive circle: The more anxious we are about being perfect, the more tense we become and the less well we are able to function, which in turn proves how worthless we are! This pattern can undermine our work and our relations with others, and it is always a part of sexual inadequacy. The more we look on and worry about how we are doing, the less we are involved in a whole and satisfying way.

Another destructive must is the thought that we *must* be liked, loved, or approved of by other people—or else we are worthless. This fearful preoccupation with others' opinions promotes anxiety, tension, and egocentricity. It is desirable and pleasant to be liked and loved. But it is not necessary. The only person one must be accepted by is oneself, and by working to get out of our fearful, egoistic state (by centering and meditation) we can gradually feel good about ourselves. Then, in a healthy state of Self, (see the Personality Chart) we will be more lovable, but this will no longer be a matter of urgency. Only then will we be like a tree with roots, rather than like a leaf blown by the wind in every direction.

Another must is the compulsion to be better than others in whatever we do. We all have our strengths and weaknesses. When we focus on developing ourselves for the satisfaction of personal growth, rather than to be superior to others, our energies can be used constructively. We become grateful for the gift of life and conscious of being a part of the Life Force, rather than worrying about being better than others while trapped in our anxious egos.

What Ifs

Life has its uncertainties, and there are no guarantees of anything. Who can be certain that today is not our last day of life? When we are healthily involved in living, creating, enjoying, growing, and loving, there is no energy available for worried and anxious thinking. When we are caught in our little egos, however, there is no end to our doubts and fears.

Instead of being alive in the here and now, *what-if thinking* is constantly concerned about the terrible things that could happen. Most of them never happen, and when they do they are often blessings in disguise or opportunities for growth. The only finality is death, and then our problems are over. Worries such as what if "I fail," "I lose my job," "I make a mistake," "I am rejected," "I get nervous," "I look foolish," and so on must be seen as a waste of energy and source of tension and anxiety. We can eliminate them by constantly challenging them with rational thinking and by working with the positive techniques introduced in this book. Centering awareness on the point below your navel and feeling your weight underneath can help you "settle down" in any situation and think more reasonably at any moment of your life (see page 244, Aikido).

Distorted Thoughts

We often tell ourselves lies and half-truths. Demosthenes, the Greek philosopher, was aware of this tendency: "Nothing is so easy as to deceive one's self; for what we wish, we readily believe." We may, for example, tell ourselves that other people are responsible for our unhappiness. Self-pitying people can spend years in psychoanalysis, but they continue to make themselves unhappy through their own attitudes and behavior. Do you blame the world instead of realizing that, if you are being mistreated, it is your problem, your creation, and your responsibility? Only by facing this truth can you take steps toward constructive change and growth. The alternative is martyrdom, misery, and "woe is me."

Another common self-deception is the idea that it is easier to keep our neurotic patterns than struggle to overcome them. People often allow their inner fears to keep them rationalizing in this fashion until a crisis occurs and their illusions and defenses break down. At this point, some individuals adopt more overt defenses, such as drug or alcohol addiction. Changing old attitudes takes work and faith, but success is well worth it. So counter this self-defeating thought with the fact that growing pains are better than dying pains. Visualize the person you wish to be; then use our Syntonic techniques to be your real Self.

A third distorted idea is that things should always go well, and if they don't, life is terrible. The bitter and the sweet are both parts of reality. If you make the best of problems, they are opportunities for growth. If you dwell on how terrible your problems are, you will have the meager satisfaction of feeling sorry for yourself and boring everyone who listens to you. There is a prayer that everyone might use daily and take to heart: "God, give me the strength to change what I cannot accept, to accept that I cannot change, and the wisdom to distinguish between the two." I forget who created it but the prayer is unforgetable!

Fourth, challenge the distorted thought that because you had a difficult past you must inevitably continue to suffer!

By all means, face the past that you are carrying around in yourself today in your tensions and attitudes (the negative inner child and parents). Also list the good things you enjoyed then and the positive qualities you have now. Then challenge the qualities you want to eliminate, and use the release techniques and positive imagery of Syntonic therapy. As the philosopher George Santayana said in a lecture at Harvard: "He who does not learn from the past is doomed to repeat it."

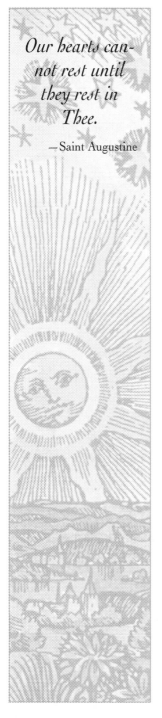

Our hearts cannot rest until they rest in Thee.

—Saint Augustine

FOURTEEN

Improve Your Spiritual Health

Humans have always been in awe of the cosmic mystery in which they find themselves. With knowledge, fear is replaced by respect for the awesome creativity and integrity of the universe. Democritus wrote, "Of the many wonders that be, there is none more wonderful than man." This is true of humans in syntony with themselves and the order of nature, in a state of health and harmony. Out of tune with nature, however, humans are tragic rather than inspiring.

To appreciate the miracle of life, one need only contemplate how a human being is created from one cell to trillions of cells. A life lived with an attitude of reverence is the mark of a mature human being. One such man, Anaximander, lived in the sixth century B.C. He was conscious of the cosmic energy: "Air is the creative substance of all matter. The essence of the universe is in the infinite air, in eternal movement, which contains All in itself."

In India, teachers of higher consciousness called this cosmic energy Brahman, the infinite creative power of reality. The manifestation of that power in humans they named Atman. Realizing the essential unity underlying all things, they taught that Brahman (God) and Atman (the soul) are One.

Balance—The Key to Life

An essential part of wholeness is balance. All things contain a centrifugal and a centripedal force—the tendency to expand or spread out, and the tendency to hold together. If the universe were not perfectly balanced between these two complementary forces, it would fly apart or squeeze together, would it not?

The expansive tendency, called *yin* in China, is found, for example, in the idea of social freedom; while the force of order, or *yang*, is the requirement of justice. The healthy society strives for freedom and justice, which requires a constant balancing of these two forces. Unbounded freedom results in anarchy and chaos; excessive rigidity leads to stagnation.

The same law applies to humans. To be too passive is as undesirable and ineffectual as to be too aggressive. To be predominantly one or another, too *yin* or too *yang* is to be unbalanced. But balancing is not something we do with effort or will (i.e., by "looking on," or observing ourselves). For in looking on we become top heavy and lose our balance. All we can do is remove the obstacles in our bodies, emotions, and minds to uncover what has been there all along— that way of being which is our essential Self in balance with the whole, the cosmic energy that is in and through all things (see the comments on aikido on pages 190—192).

In Japan this cosmic energy is called *ki.* Koichi Tohei said, "The basic entity is One. The universe is One. A man is One. Even if you reduce it by half infinitely it never becomes zero. *Ki* is the basic unit of the universe and everything is ultimately composed of *Ki.*" (*Ki Sayings)* [1]

Energy underlies all material reality in the universe. To have health is to know how to tap and generate this internal energy. When one flows with positive *ki,* one enjoys good physical, emotional, mental, and spiritual health. When this energy is blocked by wrong living, negative *ki* causes imbalances on all levels: disturbed blood pressure, body weight, temperature; withdrawal or aggression; compulsive thinking, worthlessness, or arrogance.

Balance is really as simple as it is natural, when one understands the laws associated with it. For example, until one finds the way to balance in harmony, standing on one's head is impossible. The ways of *ki* are as simple as the flight of a bird, the swimming of a fish, or the movement of a blossoming branch in a gentle breeze. Once we clean out toxic elements which cloud our bodies and minds, light dawns. The four rules of aikido on pages 191—192 are simple but not easy. Can you look at anything for one minute without

---

[1] Op. cit. p. 190-191.

your mind jumping about? Can you relax completely without holding tension in some part of your body for one minute? Can you stand with your awareness centered in your hara, just below your navel? Can you direct your inner life force out from your body in whatever direction and to whatever distance you wish? Practicing these exercises will help you correct imbalances and increase your well-being.

Many of us occasionally catch ourselves in such a balanced state. The intermediate golfer or tennis player can make a great shot by chance, when everything comes together and it "just happens." One who is master of oneself is aware of and harmonious with nature, able to receive and extend energy effortlessly. Pro golfers are single-minded when confronting the ball; their body moves in a relaxed manner, their weight is grounded, and they follow through the ball.

In spiritual terms, when I am in the flow I am, in the words of Tagore, with the "life of my life." I am completely immersed in what I am doing. In going beyond our separate ego, we find our Self. The four dimensions of the state of Self (described in the Personality Chart) are identical with the four rules of the positive *ki* energy flow.

If you relax and intently study a flower, directing your energy outward, you are suddenly no longer "you" in your illusory cocoon of separateness but, like a butterfly dancing in the air, you are at one with the flower.

There is a story in Hindu mythology of the goddess Devi, who had found this state of enlightenment.[2] To help others find the way, she asked Shiva (the masculine principal of the Hindu trinity, Brahman, Vishnu, and Shiva) the following:

---

[2] W. O'Flaherty, *Shiva: The Erotic Ascetic*, Oxford Publishers, New York, 1973.

"O Shiva, what is your reality?
What is this wonder-filled universe?
What constitutes seed?
Who centers the universal wheel?
What is this life beyond form pervading forms?
How may we enter it fully, above space and time, names and descriptions?
Let my doubts be cleared!"

Shiva replies with 112 ways, among them my favorites are the following:

"Consider your essence as light rays rising from center to center, up your vertebrae, and so rises *livingness* in you."
After each reply, write your commentary and then compare with mine, as a metaphysical game to play together!
Commentary: [You *are energy*, beneath your transitory and evanescent form. The more you see yourself in this way, the less attached you are to your body, the more you will realize the energy that runs through the world and built our bodies.]
"Attention between eyebrows, let mind be before thought. Let form fill with breath-essence to the top of the head, and there *shower as light*."
Commentary: [When we empty our mind of thought and experience cosmic energy flowing up through our form, we bring the bliss of cosmic consciousness.]
"Eyes, closed, see your inner being in detail. Thus *see* your true nature."
Commentary: [In seeing deeply into yourself, you see that you are dancing particles.]
"Closing the seven openings of your head with your hands, a space between your eyes becomes *all inclusive*."
Commentary: [Closing your senses to the world of forms and illusions, you reach the essential wholeness of reality.]
"Feel your substance, bones, flesh, blood saturated with *cosmic essence*."

Commentary: [Open your "sixth sense" to the omni-present cosmic energy.]

"When in worldly activity, keep attentive between the two breaths, and so practicing, in a few days *be born anew.*"

Commentary: [Be in the world of forms and participate fully, but realize that all forms, including your own, change. Then be happily with Oneness.]

"Focus on fire rising up through your form from the toes up until the body burns to ashes *but not you.*"

Commentary: [You are more than your body, which is only a temporary abode for your soul or Self.]

"When some desire comes, consider it. Then, suddenly, *quit it.*"

Commentary: [Have your desires, but do not let your desires have you. Rather than being a blindly conditioned, addicted animal, practice being free from your usual habits. Be in the space between pleasure and pain; thus you can enjoy one, avoid the other, and be bound to neither.]

"Toss attachment for body aside, realizing *I am everywhere. One who is everywhere is joyous.*"

Commentary: [Egocentricity, the illusion of separateness, is like the fear of a child in the darkness. Being one's Self, one unites with the cosmic energy.]

"The appreciation of objects and subjects is the same for an enlightened as for an unenlightened person. The former has one greatness: he remains in the *subjective mood,* not lost in things."

Commentary: [In the ego we are attached to things. Anxiously trying to get them, we lose our Self. Happiness is being in the world but not of it.]

"Feel the consciousness of each person as your own con-sciousness. So, leaving aside concern for self, *become each being.*"

Commentary: [Melt the anxiousness that keeps you imprisoned in your ego and separates you from loving others and your Self as part of the cosmic energy. Practice this empathy as you breathe in your center and emerge from the darkness of your egotism.]

Meditation Techniques to Experience Cosmic Energy

Optimal health is gained by learning to be in accord with the laws of nature. In the spiritual dimension, this means being aware that we are created as manifestations of the cosmic energy, and experiencing ourselves in relation to the power in and around us. In theological language, this has been called "practicing the presence of God" in which "we live and move and have our being." Various ways have been devised to still the chatter of the ego-mind, and to discover the blissful silence of the soul or Self.

Using Sounds for Inner Peace and Healing

Sounds, like everything in the universe, are made of energy vibrations. The more we feel those vibrations, the more alive we are and the greater our contact with the Life Force. The ancient sages who explored the inner universe found the sound "Ohhhhhhhmmmmmmmmmmmm" to be in harmony with cosmic vibration.

Sitting comfortably upright, inhale through your nose sharply and deeply to engage your diaphragm and expand your lungs. As you exhale, make the sound "Oh," starting somewhat sharply. Gradually, closing your lips, proceed to the sound "mmmmmmmmm." Curl your tongue back at this point, and you will feel more energy building within.

Direct that energy to any part of your body by thinking of it moving there. Energy follows thought; you can use this inner power to help heal or revitalize various parts of your body.

A second exercise is as follows: Sitting comfortably upright, or lying down on a flat surface, fold your fingers over your forehead and gently close your ears with your thumbs. You can do this by sliding your thumbs toward your ears and inserting them into your ears, as if to close off outside sounds.

Listen to the inner sound. Concentrate on it completely and let it permeate your consciousness. Let it quiet all activity of your mind so that no "records" are playing. Breathe gently and easily into your center and melt into this inner sound. It may remind you of the sound in a conch shell held to your ear. Feel its depth and spend several minutes as a "wireless receiver" of this manifestation of the cosmic energy within and around you.

The more you clear your mind, the more you will be master rather than slave of the mental part of your being. Gradually you will be free to think or *not* to think. Through this exercise, you will be able to experience the spiritual dimension of your essential Self. Allow your body to relax as the sound permeates your being, and you will experience "the peace that passeth understanding." (Philippians 4:7)

In a lecture at Amherst College, Albert North Whitehead defined religion as "what a man does with his aloneness." Although too narrow for my liking, this definition catches a spiritual truth. When we are alone and are tuned in to the cosmic energy around us, we enjoy the fullness of solitude. In this state, we are serene in our soul. I have known many joyful moments in this state. When we are tuned out, however, aloneness becomes loneliness and alienation. In a state of fear, our energy withdraws and we lose awareness of our connection with our Creator. The exercises give us the freedom to choose serenity or dis-ease!

A third spiritual exercise helps expand your energy field and overcome unrest. Discard your shoes, and feel your feet making contact with the floor while sitting comfortably erect. Place your hands palm upward on your knees; close your eyes and focus on gently breathing into your abdomen. Feel the breath very gently expand your ribs and chest. Feel a slight lifting up as you breathe in, and a relaxed settling down as you exhale. Feel the gentle rise and fall of your shoulders.

Now listen for the inmost sound, and gradually you will become aware of a rich, full silence, beyond all sound. Surrender to the peace and quietness of that silence. Let yourself be one with that silence. As you return to your ordinary state, you will have an awareness of wholeness and cosmic consciousness. Your body will be relaxed, your mind clearer. The great teachers instruct that no matter how stormy the surface of the ocean, there is peace and syntony in the depths. While in this state we are "in the world"—yet we have a security that can come only when in touch with the Cosmic Force. Thus, we are not "of the world"; the importance of things and people falls into place in proper proportion. The Buddha said, "The man who cannot be happy with nothing, cannot be happy with everything."

Meditation with Movements

Sitting comfortably upright, picture a plumb line coming down through your head and spine, so your head is balanced on your shoulders, neither pulled in nor too far forward. This creates a better conductor of energy flow.

Hold your left (receptive) hand palm upward on your knee. Picture energy flowing into your hand from the Life Force. Move your right hand, palm facing your body but without touching it, to any part of your body that feels tension or pain. Pain is blocked energy. Picture your hand sending energy to that area, and imagine obstructions dissolving as you breathe gently into your center.

Another exercise can be done standing, with feet about a foot apart and parallel. As you inhale, raise your arms upward and slightly apart, hands open, as if to embrace a loved one. Picture yourself receiving the cosmic energy. Holding your breath, keep that position as long as it is comfortable; and then, exhaling, let your arms come down to rest. As you are reaching out with your arms, you may think "I am." Experience the "I" in tune with the cosmic energy. As you lower your arms to rest, think, "One with life." Like a boat with a keel, you will never be swamped by the storms that may rage outside of you.

Breathing Meditation

Meditation has been defined by many people in many ways; as a way to quiet one's mind, as sustained reflection and also as the continuous application of the mind to the contemplation of some religious truth, mystery, or object of reverence. Aldous Huxley said in a lecture: "Meditation has been used in every part of the world and from the remotest periods as a method of acquiring knowledge about the essential nature of things." In its highest form, I believe meditation is the way to discover the unity of one's essence with God.

Sitting in a comfortable, upright position, close your right nostril with the thumb of your right hand, and inhale gently and deeply through your open left nostril. Close the left nostril with the index finger of the same hand, hold for a count of three, and then gently and fully exhale through the right nostril, removing your thumb. Continue this alternate breathing without strain. Feel the air going into every cell of your body. Feel the Oneness with this breath energy, for "breath is life." "And the Lord God formed man of the dust of the earth, and breathed into his nostrils the breath of life, and man became a living soul." (Genesis 2:7) Would you trade your next breath for anything else in the world?

Experiencing the Cosmic Energy

Take a comfortable position, either sitting or lying down. Open your awareness to the fact that Life Force is in and around you at all times. With your eyes closed, picture this energy coming down from the outer universe like white rays of light. Picture these rays gently penetrating your mind, and feel their warmth relaxing your brain. Imagine this healing energy burning out the old patterns and negative images that have a destructive effect on your life. Feel it melting the fear and hostility connected to these thoughts and images. Feel your mind becoming brighter and more clear and free.

Now picture this cosmic energy flowing down through every cell and organ of your body. Picture the energy of white light flowing through your face and neck and throat, through your shoulders, arms, and hands . . . feel it penetrating through your trunk and within your body . . . flowing through your pelvis, legs, ankles, and feet, and then flowing out to the world. Feel it recharge your center just below your navel, freeing tensions so that once again you can draw a free breath. Feel the white light strengthening any area of your body that needs this healing power.

Imagine this cosmic energy like a stream flowing freely down a mountainside, happily dancing through your being. Allow yourself to surrender to it and to feel like an open channel for this Life Force. In losing your ego, you will find your Self.

Now picture the Life Force flowing out lovingly from your body to heal and revitalize others—friends and loved ones. Allow it to flow out to people you fear or toward whom you feel anger, envy, or hostility. As you send healing rays toward them, you will be healing yourself of the negative emotions that damage your own body and spirit.

The more you go with the positive flow of this Life Force, the more sense of self-worth and inner freedom you will enjoy. As you give off positive vibrations, more new energy will be given to you.

For this reason, we say God is love. Love is the creative power within us. The power of love is the opposite of fear. The more we feel the flow of love, the less afraid we become. Remember the two-sided autonomic nervous system? (See the Personality Chart.) And in a state of love, we can be assertive of our own rights as well as respectful of the rights of others. When you open yourself to this state of Oneness with the Life Force, say to yourself the following: "I am. I am of value. I am worthy of loving and respecting myself, with all my limitations, because I am created by and part of the Life Force of the universe."

Another way to shift from the negative ego state to the God centered loving state which is everyone's essence, is by using the Taoist technique of "smiling energy." We are created as we have said with a dual autonomic nervous system; when we smile from our hearts the parasympathetic takes over and "casts out" the hate/fear or fight/flight system. So breathe deeply, settle down, and visualize someone or something that opens your heart with a loving smile. I think of special moments with one of my grandchildren, and I am immediately restored by the grace of God to my true and loving Self. We always have a choice and the God given freedom to be negative and petty, or positive and free!

Keys to Improving Your Spiritual Health and Vitality

- Use the "ohhhmmmmm" sound to open the energy flow.
- Empty your mind by merging with the inner sound.
- Sit upright with palms upward: Be one with your breath.
- Receive cosmic energy with your left hand and direct it with your right hand.
- Embrace the universe and become one with life.
- Recharge your batteries (glands or *chakras*) with alternate nostril breathing.
- Picture the cosmic energy healing you and others.
- The more conscious you are of your cosmic connection, the more you will be blessed with enthusiasm, which means "to be filled with the grace of God."
- If there is some fault or action that you feel guilty about, without hating or blaming yourself go beyond thought (the ego-mind in which there is no peace) and in meditation experience instant forgiveness as you reconnect with God within, the Infinite Light, and the gift of grace. Then visualize yourself as that new, free person, and then be so!
- Choose a visualization that will tap your true Self, and connect you with your smiling energy, and the kingdom of God within you. Once again you will enjoy the gift of the fruits of the Spirit, and the freedom that accompanies the Spirit. (II Corinthians 3:17)

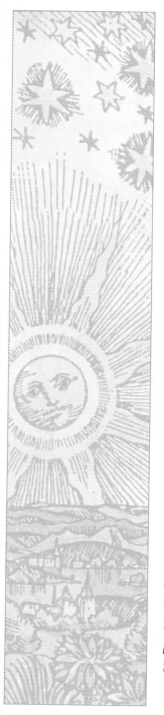

FIFTEEN

Your Greatest Opportunity for Personal Growth

It is a common human tendency to avoid or postpone facing unpleasantness. All living things, from the amoeba (that one-celled organism we learned about in biology) to humans, have this built-in resistance. Unlike other creatures, however, we have intelligence, which gives us the ability to question and choose between alternatives rather than act instinctively or automatically like roosters and red snappers. For good or ill, we have this freedom. Sometimes (when we are duped by

283

fear, greed, or short-range hedonism) our choices are disastrous. At other times, when we are clear and together, we "see
life steadily and see it whole," as Plato said if I remember my
college philosophy. Then we choose what is truly good,
though the results might not be immediately gratifying.

So my friend, before you put this book on the shelf, I
suggest you do the following. First, focus on your center
just below your navel while sitting comfortably upright.
You cannot breathe freely or be a channel for the Life
Force when you slump. Second, breathe into your whole
body and exhale toward the whole universe; feel your
weight underneath. Third, remain in this state of aware
relaxation as you answer the following questions from your
center, with body, mind, and spirit—*not with your mind alone*.
(Remember, your mind alone is a master of self-deception
and rationalization, and it replays the old records from the
past, which need to be scrapped.)

Four Key Areas for Your Personal Development

Physical Well-Being

Are you generally full of energy, enjoying all the bodily
functions you were born with, free of illnesses or symptoms
such as aches, pains, headaches, colds, etc., and able to
enjoy a relaxed body when you work or play?

If your answer is "no" and you wish to enjoy real physical health and the moment-to-moment pleasure that goes
with this state, thumb through the first section of this book
and list the things you choose to do to improve your physical well-being. Remember, you didn't get fat, tense, or worn
out in a day; so be like the tortoise who defeated the rabbit
and win the race for health in a slow but sure way.

Emotional Well-Being

Are you generally happy that you are alive, enjoying a sense of warm-heartedness that can express itself in compassion, friendliness, self-assertiveness, and love in ways appropriate to the situation? Are you able to make decisions not from fear, but through knowledge of what is best for you? Are you strong enough to take the growing pains that go with change and the uncertainty that goes with growth?

If you cannot honestly answer "yes," my friend, your emotional level of health is not what it could be. This may be due partly to physical errors in living, so list the things in Section I with which you can improve yourself, and then outline your own wholistic program as you review Section II.

Mental Well-Being

Is your mind generally bright and clear, able to think things through without self-deception, free of worry, envy, ego tripping, self-negation, grandiosity, pettiness, greed, and spite? Are you free to think or not think as you choose, so that your mind is your servant and not your master?

Your answer will probably be "no," since we rarely learn anything about *practical techniques* of mental health, even in graduate studies in clinical psychology. To get your mind straight, you cannot work with the mind alone; for where your mind stops and your body begins, no one knows. List the positive changes you decide to make from Section I, and whatever emotional release and stress reduction exercises you feel you need from Section II. Then outline the techniques you wish to practice from Section III to revise your thinking.

Spiritual Well-Being

Do you generally feel aware of a Source of your being that sustains your existence from moment to moment? Are you at one with this Life Force with every breath that brings energy flowing through you? Are you serene in your awareness of this higher power and free of the prison of egotism and vanity? Are you grateful for the miracle of creation, including yourself?

If your answer is "yes," you are far along the way toward being a whole and fulfilled person, and you are enjoying the fruits of wholistic living in Syntony with life. To experience the joy of spiritual wellness, you must also be on the healthy path in the other dimensions of your life. You cannot build a house on mud. Nor can you have a shining spirit based on a tense and mistreated body, on negative emotions, or on destructive thinking. Syntony means all four areas are in harmony.

If your answer is no, it is more than likely that the other three dimensions of your life need constructive change. How can you be right with God, or the creative force of the universe, if you are out of tune with your own body, with your Self, and with your fellow human beings?

Review each of the four parts of this book and choose from the inner wisdom of your center—not from your head alone—the things that will enrich your life in a total or wholistic way. Spell out in large letters, to put on the wall, the program *you* decide on to improve *your* life. Here is my program as an example. But you are responsible for your own. It is your life, my friend, and your decisions will determine whether it will be healthy and happy, or sick and miserable.

My Own Syntonic Program

Upon Awakening

1. If feeling anxious or tense, I practice five minutes of emotional release through spontaneous sounds and movements.
2. If necessary, I practice stamping, kicking out, or pounding with anger at the tensions that block my freedom.
3. Then I do ten minutes of alternate nostril breathing and stretching exercises, the candle, bicycle and plow. (See drawing.)
4. Then three minutes of self-reflexology.
5. Then I do the Heavenly Drum and smiling energy exercises.
6. Sitting upright and aware of my center I focus on positive imagery; I visualize myself open to the Life Force behaving in a happy and positive way during the day.
7. After a shower, and a brisk rubdown, I then practice aikido meditation ending with the "ohmmmmm" vibration.

Affirmations

My Body

I will avoid all poisons that hurt my body: nicotine, caffeine, chocolate, sugar, white flour, soda, ice cream, excessive fats, and alcohol. I will eat whole, natural foods and enjoy sports and walk for exercise whenever possible.

My Emotions

I will try to be aware at all times of my center and weight underneath, since this helps me feel relaxed and secure. I will express my positive and assertive feelings whenever possible and extend positive energy to the world.

My Mind

I will not allow negative and neurotic thoughts to control me. I will picture them as old "records" that must be broken, and I will replace them with rational and constructive thoughts. I will also practice being beyond thought, above the ego-mind, to experience the joy that accompanies the "peace that passeth understanding."

My Spirit

I will be aware of the Cosmic Power at all times so that I can be free of anxious egocentricity and grateful for the many blessings I now enjoy; to be in the world but not of it.

Upon Retiring

I will review the day and do quiet visualization and spiritual exercises like Smiling Energy before sleeping. I will do the Heavenly Drum, the gateway to meditation beyond thought, to peace and oneness.

In creating your own wholistic program, keep in mind that the best results come from making positive changes in all four dimensions of your life. If even one is forgotten, all the rest will suffer.

Remember the story of the four blind men and the elephant? Each touched a different part of the beast and insisted that *that* was the way it was. The one who touched the trunk insisted it was a great serpent; the one who touched the leg determined it was a tree trunk; and so forth.

This is the trouble with self-help psychology books, nutritional books, emotional growth manuals, or books about spiritual wisdom. All have an important part of the truth, but each neglects the other indispensable parts of the whole person.

You Have a Choice

There are two things, along with death and taxes, that you can be certain of. One is that everything changes. As Heraclitus said, "You never step into the same river twice." You cannot stay the same, and inevitably you will change toward or away from well-being.

Second, there are laws on every level of life. Whether you violate them or respect them will determine your destiny. You cannot undo your past, and if you are ill, fearful, worrisome, and out of sync, you have usually brought this state on yourself. Shakespeare put it best in Hamlet: "To suffer the slings and arrows of outrageous fortune, or take arms against a sea of troubles and by opposing, end them." If you are tired of suffering, or want greater well-being, this book has all you need to know to achieve your goal.

Deep in your center, your inner wisdom knows that the false values of possessions and social status do not lead to fulfillment, but that health, love, peace of mind, and genuine spirituality are what life is all about. True happiness appears when you live in harmony with life by being in touch with your real needs and your real Self.

When you are centered and experience this state of wholeness, you will be *free*—perhaps for the first time in your life. You will no longer *have* to have a drink, a cigarette, a sexual act, a certain number of dollars, a certain relationship; your mind will be clear of the obsessions and compulsions that have made you a slave. And no longer dependent on others for "happiness," you will not continue to let them control your life.

In your egoistic and head-dominated state, what you called love was really fearful dependency. Even if you were married to that person, you were always secretly afraid of losing what you had. But real love can only come out of inner fullness, when you are in touch with the Life Force and are independently happy with your Self. Only when you find that inner balance and harmony are you *ready* to have an authentic relationship. You cannot love and respect another person unless *you* are a person that *you* can respect and love.

As you follow the program you choose for your Self, slowly but surely you will build the health and happiness that are your birthright. However disturbed and discordant human existence is at this stage of history, when humans are still in their emotional and spiritual infancy, in your inner Self you will be in tune and send positive vibrations to the world around you. This is my wish for you, my friend. Godspeed on your journey; the adventure of fulfilling the syntony you were designed to enjoy!

Lifetime Affirmations

Here are examples of thoughts and attitudes that will strengthen and nurture your spiritual strength and well-being. You can add to them or change them as you wish, record them and play them hypnotically back to yourself after you create a deeply relaxed state within, and thereby concretize these attitudes.

I am one with the Infinite Power of the universe.

I am surrounded by peace and harmony.

I can be centered when the outer world is chaotic.

I accept God's acceptance and feel transformed.

I am free of tensions, fears, guilt feelings, and shame.

I feel the Holy Spirit with every breath.

My pleasure and joy increase as I grow spiritually.

I reject the way of contraction, fear, hate, and worry.

I choose the way of expansion, love, understanding, and faith.

The more I express love, the more good things come to me.

I am filled with light and protected by this power.

I am open to faith, hope, and love.

I am grateful for the gift of every breath and moment.

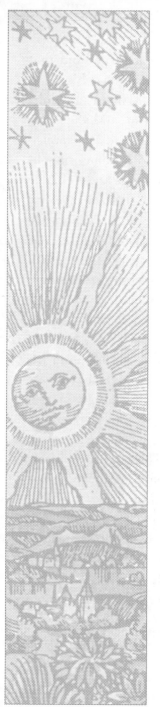

The Way to a Happy Family

Like a beautiful yacht floundering on a reef, the Culver family was grinding itself to pieces. Father was a successful plastic surgeon, mother an attractive and accomplished artist, and Tim, Donna, and David, aged thirteen, eleven, and ten, respectively, were also bright, attractive, and talented. And yet there was stark tragedy in this family, and they were finally driven to seek help and came to me for family group therapy.

Ostensibly, Tim was the problem, but it turned out that he was only the scapegoat. Father would let loose his rages on Tim and then out of guilt pamper him for a while. Mother would keep complaining about Tim, and she overlooked her self-created misery that was due to her spoiled prima donna attitudes. Donna and David became diabolically clever in learning to get away with things and to blame Tim, in a vain attempt for recognition. And Tim, in rage and despair, fought back by failing at school and desperately provoking more punishment at home. Even Raggles, the dog, could not stand the shrillness of voices, the tightness of bodies, the gracelessness of movement, and the atmosphere of desperation and hostility. Raggles would either snap, whimper, or set about gnawing the kitchen chairs.

In contrast, when I visited the Hollander family on a ski weekend in Vermont, there were musical vibrations in the atmosphere, and voices and bodies and movements were pleasant and harmonious. Orders were never given, but rather reasonable and thoughtful suggestions were made. No one was ignored, but each was respected as a person with unique interests and talents. The three children, slightly younger than those in the unhappy Culver family, enjoyed one another and showed in many little ways their mutual affection.

Dad, a man rugged enough to have built his own ski lodge, had a tender and loving touch when his children came to him. And mother, comfortable and secure in her own right, gave forth a warmth like sun streaming through stained glass windows. Everyone had a place here—everyone felt significant and respected the importance of one another. It came as no surprise to learn that once or twice a week they had a family meeting, discussed ways of solving any problems that may have arisen, and shared suggestions to improve things for everyone. I also learned that both parents were aware of the connection between nutrition and physical and emotional health. No sugar and junk food was another reason for the happy atmosphere!

The family, like a tree, is known for its fruits. There is no greater fulfillment of human life than a family in which parents and children live together in mutual love, respect, cooperation, and enjoyment. Nor is there greater misery than a family in conflict, in which the members are pitted one against the other in fear, hostility, and endless bickering.

The high incidence of unhappy or broken homes, disturbed children and adolescents, and confused parents (who carry over the destructive attitudes of their own childhood experiences) indicates a vast incompetence in parents to manage family group living. Yet how could this be otherwise? To drive a car, one must show basic knowledge and skill, or else one is not licensed to do so. The ultimate responsibility, family leadership and the raising of children, is left to chance, and the results are often disastrous.

Our family chaos is an indictment of our education on all levels. Unlike certain diseases which defy human comprehension, emotional illness is well understood. Pleasure and anxiety, love and fear, goodwill and hatred, and the conditions that create them are generally comprehended. Personality cannot grow in isolation; but whether it grows in healthy or destructive ways depends on the nature of the family group in which it is created. There is, however, a tremendous gap between our knowledge of mental health and group organization, and the application of that knowledge.

About fifty years ago at the Child Research Center of the University of Iowa, three brilliant experimental psychologists, Kurt Lewin, Ronald Lippitt, and Ralph White, conducted an experiment that proved the importance of democratic group organization for emotional health and individual productivity.[1] They trained adults in three different types of leadership: authoritarian, in which the leader as boss determined all the policies and activities of the group; laissez faire, in which the leader left the group to its own devices; and democratic, in which the leader made all policies a matter of group discussion and assisted the members of the group in making their own decisions. (In family life, these leadership types would be described as the strict parent, the overpermissive parent, and the parent who avoids either of these extremes by asserting his or her own rights and respecting the rights of the children.)

The effects of these social climates on the behavior of the ten-year-old boys in these experimental groups were significant. In terms of efficiency and productive accomplishment in painting and carpentry projects, the group with weak leadership was greatly inferior to the others. Surprisingly, the democratic group was as productive as the authoritarian one. However, the psychologists noted two other factors in favor of democracy. First, the genuine interest in work was decidedly greater in this group, since a greater amount of work-minded conversation took place, and a higher level of creativity was achieved. Second, when the adult leader left the room, the boys in the democratic group continued on their own, while in the autocratic group they stopped as if relieved of something they had to do.

For parents who want to be better parents—that is, better leaders—the emotional factors are paramount. What of love and hate, pleasure and tension, happiness and negativity?

[1] Kurt Lewin, Ronald Lippitt, and Ralph K. White, "Leader Behavior and Member Reaction in Three Social Climates," *Group Dynamics: Research and Theory*, (Third Edition), Harper & Row Pub., pp 318-335.

Which kind of leader was resented, and which kind loved? Which kind of group created mutual respect, friendliness, and cooperation, and which kind engendered hostility and scapegoating? Are not these attitudes the very fabric of mental, emotional, and family health, or sickness, as the case my be?

The results were startling: There was much more hostility (in a ratio of 30 to 1), more demands for attention, more destruction of property, and far more scapegoat behavior in the boss-led groups. Think of contemporary student behavior. (Parents note: These are all the things that make family life miserable!) On the positive side, not only did nineteen out of twenty boys feel more warmly toward their democratic leaders (no mystery, since the democratic leaders showed their affection by respecting the feelings and interests of the boys), but these groups were characterized by more friendliness, sharing, and cooperation. Since these are the values that parental common sense, clinical psychology and psychiatry, and religion espouse, what stands in our way of achieving them?

So many American parents are lost in confusion about authority and discipline. Imagine the captain of a ship who didn't know where his vessel was, nor where it was going. He might bark orders in his uncertainty, or pretend everything would be all right—or desperately alternate between those two irrational activities (which frightened parents often do). A brilliant line from a poem by W.H. Auden says "We are lecturing on navigation while the ship is going down." The real need is for a sound course of action that will get the family in a safe channel between the extreme of no discipline, on the one hand, and destructive "boss" discipline on the other.

There is an immediate solution that the average family (of normal intelligence and emotional balance) can employ *now*.

The answer is to establish a democratic atmosphere by having *family group meetings* in which each member has the right and obligation to express verbally his or her true thoughts, feelings, and suggestions. This will afford parents as well as their children an opportunity for self-expression, mutual understanding, and increasing self-respect.

In families in which discipline has been lacking, and in which the children have dominated the parents, the beleagured adults often suppress their resentment and attempt to take some control by using guilt-provoking remarks like "You'll be the death of me," or "We've sacrificed our lives for you kids." Such ineffectual and self-negating parents can learn, in democratic family meetings, to *assert themselves* and share in making family rules that are necessary for the well-being and health of all the members.

And what of families in which domineering or dictatorial discipline has reigned? In these families, scapegoating of one member, or sometimes a "pecking order" of resentment, takes place. As in all tyrannies, the choice is either to rebel or submit. Children who rebel against rules which they had no part in making act out their rightful indignation by waging guerrilla warfare against their parents, and later against society. Our prisons are overflowing! Those who submit internalize their resentment, become tense and function below par, and often spitefully "get back" by hurting themselves. Our hospitals are also overflowing!

Children with either type of reaction basically feel unloved, for love in its true sense involves a respect for the individuality of the other person. And they are right, for in a tyranny the thoughts, feelings, and values of the individual are not important!

There is no blame intended for parents who have tried either or both types of unproductive leadership. Self-blame must be regarded as a foolish waste of energy. The real fault is with our schools and colleges, in which classes are still organized in an authoritarian fashion and courses on individual happiness, personal growth and effective parenthood are usually nonexistent.[2] On a positive note, then, what can well-meaning parents do (and this includes the vast majority of parents) to make family life a rich and exciting adventure?

Six Steps Toward a Happy Family

1. Have a family group meeting, with all members from four years of age invited. Explain that at these meetings everyone will have a chance to express his or her thoughts and feelings, and together find ways to improve understanding and solve family problems. As parents, admit where you have been at fault—without self-blame (since everyone makes mistakes) but with a view toward improvement. I have often seen such truthfulness unleash the creative power of forgiveness in children and heal long-standing breaches.[3] This will also help children admit their unreasonable attitudes and behavior— in an atmosphere of rationality, where no one is expected to be perfect.[4]

---

[2] H. Giles and R. Kronemeyer, "Self-Evaluation of a Group Therapy Experience by Graduate Students and Its Implications," *The International Journal of Social Psychiatry Vol. XI, No. 3,* 1965.

[3] R. Kronemeyer, "Roots of Democracy Can Grow In Camp," *Camping Magazine,* February 1964, Vol. 36, No. 2.

[4] J. Cook, "Camp Offers Practice in Self Rule." *The New York Times.* August 27, 1964.

2. Suggest that each member have a turn to "chair" the meetings, but have the family as a whole decide on future meetings. Try to have at least two meetings per week *before* mealtime. Each family member may call a meeting when necessary. So great is the need for real communication that I have never yet known a family that did not wish to continue such meetings, once a democratic procedure was started!

3. Be patient, and remember that there are no magical transformations in human beings. Growth in all of nature is a gradual process. Often, like sap invisibly flowing before the spring bloom, creative forces of trust and honesty are at work though they are yet unseen. One family of five which had wrongly blamed and scapegoated the middle child, a fourteen-year-old boy, turned to him in a family meeting for the first time with an attitude of helpfulness. He later admitted that this was the first time he ever felt respected and cared for, and was then able to see, through eyes washed clean with tears, the ways in which he had been hurting himself and spiting others in his family.

4. Some families find that writing down agreed-on "laws" is a helpful way of keeping in mind desirable ways of behavior. Rules arrived at through discussion in which all members participate are much more likely to be understood and followed than those made in dictatorial fashion!

From 1955 to 1975 I founded and directed Camp New Horizon, a "children's democracy" in Southampton, Long Island, in which this method proved successful. The daily group meetings afforded children an opportunity for self-expression, self-discipline, and self-understanding. The former president of the American Group Therapy Association, Dr. Milton Berger, visited this democracy in action and wrote the following for our brochure: "Your daily group meetings are both unique and significant. In a setting free from fear, guilt and blame, you encourage honest self-expression and allow children to be authentic . . . to learn to manage their own feelings and improve their relationships with others . . . to grow in self-esteem and to develop more positive ways of being." These same principles hold true in the democratic family group as well.

5. When a group member brings up a problem and his or her feelings about it, try to empathize by putting yourself in his or her shoes (i.e., "You feel hurt, angry, sad, disappointed, etc. whenever . . ."). This will help the person become more real and honest and release inner tension, and will lead to closeness, trust, and mutuality. This is a cardinal principle of counseling and psychotherapy and is necessary for emotional growth. Conversely, avoid name calling or blaming someone for his or her feelings: "You're a baby"; "That's stupid"; "You'll never grow up." Such personal attacks are counterproductive and lead to more hurt, defensiveness, spite, and hostility. A great deal of delinquent behavior in school and society, as well as adult criminality, stems from family-generated pain and hatred!

Most parents are still not trained to be effective democratic leaders, and with good intentions they pass on the mistakes of their permissive and/or dictatorial parents. Dr. Thomas Gordon's PET (Parent

Effectiveness Training) offers an important program to solve this problem.[5]

Dr. Gordon and I see eye to eye as you will see
from the following statement which I quote from his
book.

As a society we are employing the wrong strategies to
reduce the self-destructive and socially unacceptable behaviors of young people that occur with shocking frequency.
Our best hope of prevention is another kind of strategy —
namely, helping adults who deal with children learn new
ways to manage families, schools and youth-oriented orga-
nizations. And that strategy will require teaching adults the
skills required to govern their family, their classroom, their
group more democratically, less autocratically.

Based on my experience as a professor teaching
and counseling students at New York University, a
faculty member at The Family Institute and as a
wholistic psychotherapist with hundreds of individuals and families, I believe that Dr. Gordon is a
major voice in America today. His program (please
see in relation to Appendix IV), along with the
other aspects of syntonic education could prevent
incalcuable suffering, illness, and crime, and on the
positive side, raise the quality of life far above what
it is today.

6. Parents are individuals who do not always have to
    agree when together or in family meetings. Parents
    have feelings too, and the right to express them. "I
    feel" sentences are ways of being open and real and

---

[5] Dr. Thomas Gordon, *Teaching Children Self Discipline At Home and At School*,
Time Books, Random House, N.Y., 1989.

give other group members a clear idea of you as a person. These can range from anger, hurt, disappointment, and distrust to encouragement, trust, hopefulness, and love. In contrast to name calling (which will drive others farther away), emotional sharing often evokes caring, positive concern and new effort from others. I have often seen such emotional honesty thaw out caring and loving feelings that had been frozen by fear and spite, in parents and children.

In the family, instead of mother wielding a big stick or using the threat that "You'll be sorry when your father comes home," the suggestion that "We'll all talk it over together when Daddy comes home," is a note of rationality in a situation that could result in fear, hatred, guilt, and unhappiness for all.

In one family that put the wisdom of democracy into action, practiced democratic meetings, and became a family "indivisible, with liberty and justice for all," a twelve-year-old named Jeff put it in a nutshell: "Gosh, when everyone feels good inside, we don't even need the rules."

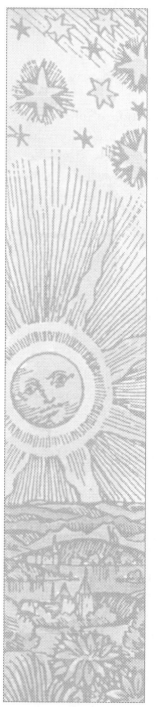

The Empathy Exercise — From Conflict to Syntony

This appendix presents a loving way to resolve misunderstandings with someone close to you. Through many years of counseling couples, I have observed that most of them would not have needed professional help if they had been able to express their feelings openly whenever the need for communication arose. By the time they come to me, of course, the grievances on both sides would fill a book, and what might have been only small skirmishes have evolved into full-scale battles.

Life is too short to waste it in wrangling, power struggles, and withdrawal. So I devised for my patients a *safe* way to talk things over. I call it the empathy exercise.

Empathy means an imaginative projection of one's own consciousness into another being, which is precisely what you do in the empathy exercise. Used correctly, it enables two people *safely* to communicate their deepest feelings, no matter what they may be, and feel closer than ever before.

Without the sharing of thoughts and feelings, a close relationship is not possible. All too often, however, one person holds back for fear of saying the wrong thing, and finally explodes when the tension can be endured no longer. Another communicates constantly in a critical way, acting out inner tensions on the hapless partner. Periods of withdrawal, bickering, and even fighting will gradually erode any relationship.

John and Kay began their married life full of hope for a happy, shared relationship. By the time their son was born, however, they were in serious trouble. Their patterns of relating, rooted in early experiences with *their* parents, soon made their home a battlefield. At this point they came to me for therapeutic help.

Kay had grown up with a distant, unloving father. Beneath her charming facade, she carried a large amount of pain and rage that she unconsciously transferred to men in general, even though she pointed to her many affairs as proof of her liking for men. These affairs had been superficial, however, and in the crucible of marriage, her deeper negative feelings inevitably surfaced. She often became, as she herself admitted, "a real bitch," who with a sneer and in a cutting voice would corner John, belittling and criticizing him.

John, on the other hand, was quiet and introspective. The child of a critical, driving, and aggressive mother, he

was, though physically powerful, a frightened and angry little boy. His pattern was to withdraw into a world of books,
safe from any human contact that might stir up his deep fear
and emotional pain. In marriage, too, he withdrew from his
painful life with Kay into a room with his books and his
computer.

For Kay, this repeated the most painful and infuriating
experience of her childhood: her father's cold indifference to
her very existence. Soon her accumulated rage spilled over
into caustic and abusive remarks, and John's desire for loving intimacy was overcome by fear and hostility.

When they came to me as a last resort before divorce,
Kay looked at John with contempt and hatred; and he was
unable to look at her at all. In couples therapy, they began
to see the ways in which they were repeating the patterns of
their unhappy childhoods, and this new awareness gradually enabled them to divert their hatred away from each
other toward its source—their primary relationships with
their parents.

At this point I introduced them to the empathy exercise,
which at first they used only during their sessions with me;
and even then, John was deathly afraid of expressing himself to Kay. When he finally took the plunge, and told her
how much her cutting remarks and criticism were hurting
him, he felt that he had made a significant step in his emotional and spiritual growth.

For the first time in his life—within the safe confines of
this simple exercise—John expressed his real thoughts and
feelings, and he found that Kay was able to accept him on a
deeper level than ever before. She began to see him not as
another cold, rejecting male, but as a human being in pain,
struggling toward freedom. The first time they did the exercise, I watched Kay's hardness melt as she saw John's inner

anguish. I asked him to risk looking into her eyes, and when he saw her warmth and compassion, his armor began to melt and he sobbed as he shared the terrible hurt of his childhood.

When they reversed roles, John found the courage to look at Kay again and enter into *her* hurt, to move out of his isolation and empathize with the pain his withdrawal had caused her. "For the first time," he said, "I was able to feel like a strong and giving man, instead of a scared and angry little boy who wanted to run away."

John and Kay set aside time every day to express their honest feelings, sharing with one another the two most important things we all need—freedom and love (that is, the chance to express ourselves honestly and freely and the healing experience of being fully accepted and deeply understood).

The empathy exercise was especially valuable for this desperate couple, but any two people in a close relationship can benefit from it. Even if you feel that you already have a completely open and honest relationship, it's possible that you simply may not be aware of what is going on inside the other person. In relationships, as in life generally, the only real security lies in dealing with what is. Using the empathy exercise will enable you to discover whether there are problems—and usually there are—and dissolve them.

Let's say that on Saturday you and your spouse went shopping for a new rug. Instead of talking out your ideas and setting a budget ahead of time, you arrived at a hostile impasse after you were in the store, and when your spouse insisted on buying the less expensive carpet, you felt hurt and put down. The result: Saturday evening you were furious but ashamed or afraid to express your anger and brooding. Or, alternatively, you actually said what was on your mind, but in such a hostile way that your spouse began to feel abused and aggrieved. Either way, it makes for an unpleasant evening, a lonely night, and a miserable Sunday. Even if you swallow your resentment to smooth things over, there is a rift in your relationship that was not there before—and it no longer has much to do with buying a rug.

A situation like the one just described is a good time for the empathy exercise. Here are the rules, which *must* be followed:

1. Either person may initiate the exercise, and the other must agree to participate. If the person does not care to, why are you with them?

2. An unpressured, private time must be set aside, when neither of you is overtired or hungry.

3. You are allowed to talk with the *guarantee* that you will not be ridiculed or sneered at.

4. Your spouse[1] or friend must really listen and enter into *your* feelings without trying to build a defense; that is, he or she must *empathize.*

5. As you pause after each positive or negative feeling you express, your spouse repeats to you as accurately and empathetically as possible the substance of what he or she understands to be your feelings, *without defending himself or herself or making accusations or excuses.* Part of the healing comes from hearing the other person give back what you have said. It is more important to feel that we are understood completely than to be agreed with.

6. When you have said all you have to say and are sure that your spouse has understood it, it's the other

---

[1] Marriage is not a prerequisite for the empathy exercise. As I stated earlier, this exercise is beneficial for any two people in a close relationship.

person's turn, and you must now *put aside your own ego* and interests to listen fully to him or her.

7. Then you must reflect back to the other person the feelings he or she has expressed to you, and so on, with your spouse talking and you responding empathetically until the air is clear. If you have been open and empathetic, you will feel closer and more trusting than you would have thought possible before you started the healing process.

Take a look at the following example:

Wife: I was really disturbed by the way you acted in the carpet store on Saturday. I felt that you were really rude to me and ignored my opinions about the rug we should have. We both earned the money to pay for it and we both have to live with it. I feel you showed a lack of respect for my desires and a real lack of respect for me as a person, and that hurts me and makes me very mad.

I feel it is important for us to at least be loyal to each other in public. Maybe the rug I wanted was a little impractical and too expensive, but it really got to me when you attacked me in front of the salesman, as if you cared more for his opinion of you than you cared for me.

Spouse: (empathizing) You really were disturbed by what I said in the carpet store and by the way I said it. You thought that I cared more for the saleman's opinion than I did for you, and you feel that my talking the way I did showed that I don't respect you or feel loyal, and that I really took advantage of you by showing lack of respect for your views in public.

Wife: Yes, and I am also hurt that you feel that your taste should prevail over mine, even though both of us are paying for the rug and both of us will be using it.

Spouse: (empathizing) You are hurt that I feel my taste should overrule yours, even though both of us are paying for the rug and both of us will be using it.

Wife: Right.

Spouse: (empathizing) Okay. It's clear we should have waited to make a decision or have tried to make a compromise. Anything else?

Wife: Well, I felt that you were very cold to me on Sunday . . . and that hurt me, too, and made me feel like you had turned against me.

Spouse: (empathizing) You felt that I was cold to you on Sunday . . . and that hurt you and made you feel that I turned against you.

Wife: Right.

Spouse: My turn?

Wife: Yes. I can breathe easier now. You go ahead with your feelings. (Note her relief from tension and more positive attitude)

Spouse: Well, the reason I was concerned about the price of the carpet and insisted on the cheaper one was because, you know, you did insist on going overboard when we got the kitchen tiles. I gave in to you on that when I felt I should not have. I felt it was my turn to make a decision and I wanted to get us out of there without running up more charges, although I agree that I should not have been rude in front of the salesman.

Wife: You felt that you had to insist on the cheaper carpet because we couldn't really afford the one I

liked and also because you felt that it was your
turn to make a household decision.

Spouse: Exactly.

Wife: And you feel that I am selfish and extravagant for
wanting to spend more than we can afford.

Spouse: No, not selfish, just thoughtless.

Wife: Okay, just thoughtless. And when I did insist on
the expensive one, you felt that I had made a one-
person decision, as I did with the tiles, and that
made you mad, and you just wanted to get out of
there without any more major expense. And that's
why you were rude.

Spouse: Yes. I felt you were trying to get me to go against
my own judgment, and really against your own
judgment, too, in buying something so out of line
with what we can afford. Budgeting is a shared
responsibility, too.

Wife: You felt I was trying to get you to go against your
own common sense . . . you felt like the grownup
taking the whole responsibility of keeping track of
our finances, especially as I had already blown the
budget on the kitchen tiles.

Spouse: Exactly. (really feels accepted and understood)

Wife: And you felt it was disloyal of me to try to manipulate you just like I felt it was disloyal of you to be
rude to me.

Spouse: Yes . . . and as for me being cold on Sunday, I
didn't feel cold so much as I felt rejected, because
when we made love Saturday night, it seemed like
you really didn't want to, but wouldn't say so.
That hurt, because it felt like you were punishing
me for doing what really was right. And when you
were so uninvolved in making love, I felt really

rejected, like you were bringing the rug problem into a place where it didn't belong.

Wife: Okay, I do understand. You felt I was punishing you for doing what really was best for us by bringing the rug problem where it didn't belong. You felt like you used to when your mom turned cold when she wanted to punish you for something. Right?

Spouse: Yes.

Wife: You are right. I was too angry to make love. We should have had this discussion on Saturday night instead of four days later. You feel, as I also feel about you sometimes, that I make one-way decisions about things that affect both of us. Neither one of us always respects the other's views and rights. [*Note:* The avoidance of airing these feelings Saturday night was caused by the fear that "opening up" would lead to more hurt and isolation.]

Spouse: I agree. But I want you to know that whatever I do, even though it might seem otherwise, I am always trying to do it for both of us.

Wife: You want me to know that whatever you do, no matter how it looks, you are doing it for both of us.

Spouse: Yes. I feel absolutely loyal to you. I do respect you. I love you.

Wife: Oh God, now I feel my heart is open to you and it feels so wonderful. Hold me close; I love you too.

This is an example of how the empathy exercise can be used to resolve the misunderstandings that arise in even the best relationships—between mates, between parents and children, between friend and friend.

It is essential to allow sufficient time and privacy, so that there is real honesty on the part of the speaker and real empathy on the part of the listener. If you both stick with the discussion until everything has been aired—and it might include some surprises that neither of you had been aware of—you'll discover that your self-respect, your respect for your partner, and your mutual trust will put down deeper and stronger roots. To communicate in this total way is to show caring in the most immediate and intimate sense. "The truth will set you free" and "Love casts out fear": In this wisdom resides the awesome power of empathy.

Most people find it hard to express their *positive* feelings of admiration, trust, respect, and love. Raised in families in which such feelings were either absent or never verbalized, we have to learn as adults to do this. The best way to free ourselves from the fear and generalized anxiety associated with positive feelings—as well as negative ones—is to risk expressing them, and the empathy exercise provides a safe environment for doing so!

Half the marriages entered into fail, and many of the others merely survive rather than grow and flower. The empathy exercise, practiced faithfully, will help destroy the weeds of distrust, fear, excessive anger and sensitivity, spitefulness, and arrogance that our inner child so often carries over into adulthood. It will also encourage the flowering of trust and respect (for oneself and the other), that is the essence of love. Empathic communication provides the rich soil, sun, and water that the tender shoots of a growing relationship need. I guarantee the effort involved in cultivating your own relationships through the empathy exercise will be richly rewarded!

Miracle Nutrients to Prevent Disease and Enhance Health

Raw Fruits and Vegetables

At least one third of your food intake should be raw. Living foods contain enzymes, vitamins, and minerals that are damaged or destroyed by cooking. Have raw fruits for breakfast before your coffee substitute or herb or green tea and your whole grain toast with apple or sesame butter. One day a week, have only fruits and salads and give your body and spirit a treat. Think prevention! Invest in organic produce or raise it or sprout it yourself!

Onions and Garlic

Although capable of sabotaging a romantic interlude, these powerful nutrients can also help reduce heart disease since they lower the tendency of the blood to clot and raise the levels of desirable high-density lipoprotein (HDL). Garlic can be taken raw in perles (sold in health stores), can lower cholesterol, and can also help clean your system of various contaminants—including parasites, which are usually picked up in traveling in more backward countries. Kyolic aged garlic is odor-free.

Flax Seed Oil

This omega 3 oil has been used widely in Europe due to the work of Dr. Johanna Budwig, who found a relationship between the unsaturated fatty acids found in linseeds (flax) and cancer prevention. On ski trips to Europe, I used to wonder why those little brown seeds were on the breakfast buffet. Buy the Omegaflo™ brand in health stores to get a quality product. Avoid hydrogenated fats (margarine) and processed oils, which are chemically altered and damaging to the body. Use flax oil or virgin olive oil on your toast. I love salad dressing made with flax oil and apple cider vinegar, and I make sure that I take two tablespoons of flax Omegaflo™ oil each day.

Soy Products and Miso Soup

The discovery of genistein in Japan, a substance that blocks the growth of new blood vessels (and therefore the growth of cancerous tumors) is focusing attention on soy products and miso soup. Along with brown rice and sea vegetables, they were part of the ancient Japanese diet of health and longevity. (Long-lived peoples have always been vegetarian rather than carnivorous.) Cabbage, brussel sprouts, and kale also have this anticancer effect.[1]

Sunflower and Pumpkin Seeds

Raw seeds have the very spark of life in them. Sprout them and you will see the miracle unfold before your eyes, In oatmeal or sugar-free granola, these seeds (along with fruit, lecithin granules, and brewer's yeast with skim milk or juice) make a healthful breakfast. Research at the Max Planck Institute in Germany has shown that many vegetable protein foods are "just as good or better than animal proteins." (Animal foods contain saturated fat and lack essential fiber as well.) Vegetable foods said to be complete proteins include soybeans, almonds, sunflower seeds, pumpkin seeds, potatoes, and all leafy green vegetables. Seeds also contain B complex vitamins, vitamins A, D, and E, zinc, phosphorus, calcium, iron, other minerals, and unsaturated fatty acids. Ask for organically raised foods and join the movement for a healthier America.

Seafoods

These foods are sources of complete protein, iodine, potassium, and polyunsaturated fatty acids. If taken from clean waters, they are more desirable than meat, which contains saturated fat and twenty-two times more phosphorus than calcium. Thus, meat eating can result in deficiencies of

---

[1] *The New York Times*[cfn], April 13, 1993.

calcium and magnesium, which can contribute to heart disease. High-fat fish like salmon, mackerel, and trout are rich sources of vitamins A and D and heart-friendly essential fatty acids.

Whole Grains

At the turn of the century, before the "advances" in milling techniques, stoneground flour contained all the nutrients and fiber of the grains, and bread was really the "staff of life." At that time, heart disease was hardly known. Today, partly because of decades of white flour use, (along with two other poisons to the body, white sugar and superheated vegetable oils and margarine), the cancer death rate is one in five and the death rate from heart disease is one in two. For sustained energy (instead of the ups and downs caused by refined sugar and flour), eat whole, natural brown rice, oats, barley, millet, and wheat. These complex carbohydrates are delicious and full of nutrients: B vitamins, vitamin E, protein, unsaturated fatty acids, iron, and other minerals. This kind of real food can prevent and cure a host of ailments that plague our society by building the immune system (e.g., colds, allergies, weight problems, hypoglycemia, diabetes, anemia, arthritis, nutritionally based mental disorders, heart problems, and cancer).

Kelp

Minerals and trace minerals from the sea are valuable and necessary nutrients for health and vitality. Minerals have the power to rejuvenate energy and to improve thinking and memory. They aid nerve impulse transmission and muscle contraction and help strengthen the nervous and skeletal systems. Health food stores carry various types of seaweeds. I also use a large shaker of kelp granules (sold by Parkelp and available at health food stores in eight-ounce jars).

Pure Water

I buy spring water drawn from areas far from chemical or industrial pollution. Distilled water is also an alternative. When I drink this, however, I make sure that I take kelp and chelated minerals for distilled water has no minerals.

Brewer's Yeast

This is a prime source of the all-important B vitamins, which are so lacking in white flour and are destroyed by the use of white sugar. There is much research on the mental, emotional, and behavioral disturbances caused by vitamin B deficiency, especially in patients troubled by anxiety and disturbed moods. In the total Syntonic approach, checking for vitamin B deficiency is necessary before one works on psychological and emotional levels. This is especially true for adolescents, who often consume a lot of junk food and sugar-laden drinks that deplete their B vitamins and add to their problems. A one-pound can of brewer's yeast (available from Lewis Laboratories) sells for under $8. I add brewer's yeast to my cereal, and it is delicious and highly nutritious.

Vitamins

If you eliminate junk food from your diet (white flour, white sugar, sodas, white rice, processed and canned foods, processed oils and margarine) and eat whole and natural grains, sprouted seeds (the best of all) raw vegetables and

fruits, and fresh seafood, you will be on the way to getting
your necessary vitamins and minerals. It is wise, however,
to enhance your diet with a quality supplement since our
foods are often depleted by growing and handling methods.
For vitamins and supplements I recommend in New York
The Atkins Center, and on the West Coast, The Staff of
Life, 509-738-2345.

Vitamin C is essential. Did you know that most mammals
produce five to ten grams of vitamin C per day, except
humans and the guinea pig? Drs. Matthias Rath and Nobel
Laureate Linus Pauling recently published their finding
that the primary cause of cardiovascular disease is a deficiency of vitamin C, which leads to the deposit of lipoprotein (a) and fibrin in the vascular wall.[2]

Heart disease is the number-one killer in the United
States. However, Drs. Rath and Pauling state that "we can
now explain why the strongest downward trend in CVD
[cardiovascular disease] mortality of all industrialized countries occurred in the USA, the country with the highest vitamin C consumption." (If you want to read more about
Rath and Pauling's research, send a contribution to the
Linus Pauling Institute of Science and Medicine, 440 Page
Mill Road, Palo Alto, CA 94306, and request their exciting
literature.) Make sure you take at least five grams of vitamin C spread out during the day. It is wise to build up to
this amount gradually if you are just beginning.

Two of my favorite nutritional physicians — Dr. Azim
Etemadi of the "Body-Mind" TV program in New York

---

2 Dr. Matthias Rath and Dr. Linus Pauling, Solution to the Puzzle of Human
Cardiovascular Disease: Its Primary Cause is Ascorbate Deficiency Leading
to the Deposition of Lipoprotein (a) and Fibrinogen/Fibrin in the Vascular
Wall. Linus Pauling Inst. of Science and Medicine, Palo Alto, CA 94306.

City and Dr. Julian Whitaker of the *Health and Healing* newsletter also recommend a daily intake of 4 or 5 grams of vitamin C, 800 to 1,200 units of vitamin E, 1,000 mg of calcium, at least 1,000 mg of magnesium, and a fish oil supplement (two to three capsules a day or more for patients with heart or lipid problems, under the care of a nutritional physician).

You may want to consult a nutritional physician for his or her own expert guidance on the use of vitamin and mineral supplements. You can write to the American Wholistic Medical Association, 4101 Lake Boone Trail, Suite 201, Raleigh, NC 27607. For $5 they will provide a list of practitioners in the state(s) of your choice.

Psyllium Husks Powder

For improved regularity and easier and more efficient elimination, this product is unexcelled. It is said that "death begins in the colon," and many doctors believe that a large percentage of all diseases orginate there and result from the stagnation of waste products. It is alimentary, my dear Watson, is it not, that the slower the transit time of waste matter, the greater the likelihood of auto-toxemia?

As many as 100 million Americans suffer from digestive diseases, from constipation to colon cancer (second as a killer only to lung cancer), at an estimated total cost of over $50 billion per year. If you are on the prudent high-fiber diet described in these pages, you will avoid being one or these tragic statistics. *You will be taking personal responsibility for your life, the real health revolution of this century! Combined with the syntonic techniques in this book to improve your emotional, mental and spiritual health, you will also enjoy a healthier, longer, and happier life in harmony with the order of the universe.*

To be on the safe side and give my system extra fiber, I use a heaping teaspoon of psyllium powder (it costs about $8 for twelve ounces and is available in health food stores) each morning in a cup of spring water or juice. For vegetable enzymes, take a Quadra-zyme Plus capsule before each meal.

If your system is functioning naturally, you will have two to three bowel movements each day. Along with no smoking, daily exercise, and a good-quality vitamin-mineral supplement, this regimen will give you a solid foundation on which to build emotional, mental, and spiritual health! Always remember: The best combination is a sound mind in a sound body, and "the body is the temple of the spirit."

Tea for Two—and For Health

I have always enjoyed Green Tea, but I was amazed when a research update from the Life Extension Institute of which I am a member (I hope it works; so far, so good) described it as "one of the most potent disease-preventing substances known. Green teas wide range of health benefits include reductions in the risk of heart disease, stroke, cancer and viral-bacterial infections. In antioxidant studies, Green Tea extracts were 200 times more potent than vitamin E in inhibiting lipid peroxidation in the brain."[3]

Epidemiological studies go on to show, according to this report which is based upon "100 scientific papers," a lower rate of cancer in regions where Green Tea was consumed. Similar dietary surveys in Japan showed a much lower incidence of stomach, liver, pancreatic, breast, lung, and skin cancers. With animals bred to develop cancer, Green Tea in

---

[3] Life Extension Update, Vol. 5, No. 1, Jan 1992.

some studies prevented cancer altogether. At Rutgers University, animals given Green Tea ten days before exposure to ultra violet light developed 50% fewer skin cancers. According to Allan H. Conner, the study director, "There aren't many things that have as broad a spectrum as Green Tea." Since today's cancer epidemic is the result of exposure to natural carcinogens such as UV sunlight, and synthetic ones such as pesticides, white sugar, margarine, processed and chemicalized, pasteurized and over cooked and enzymeless dead foods, Green Tea offers some protection against them. Of course first eliminate the ones you can.

As if this was not enough, Green Tea is also a potent ally against heart disease. It inhibits platelet aggregation that cause blood clots, heart attacks and strokes. It also reduces cholesterol, can lower blood pressure by inhibiting the angiotension-converting enzyme (ACE). Thus you may not need the drugs that work the same way *but* with side effects! It also acts to inhibit the oxidation of LDL (the "bad" cholesterol) within the arterial wall if, as just mentioned in the Linus Pauling research, the wall is vulnerable due to a lack of vitamin C.

Furthermore, Green Tea has been shown to have an anti-viral effect on the influenza virus, an anti-bacterial effect on microbes involved in food poisoning and in dental plaque, dental caries and gingivitis, as well as the positive effect of lowering blood sugar levels and a beneficial lessening of insulin levels.

Lecithin

This substance is made from soybeans and is needed by every living cell in the human body. Cell membranes, which determine which nutrients enter or leave each cell are mainly composed of lecithin without which these membranes would harden. As one gets older this supplement is essential to help prevent hardening of these membranes, increase brain function, repair damage to the liver caused by alcohol, and increase energy. Those with high serum cholesterol should take it to protect organs and arteries from fatty build-up.

The Solgar brand lecithin granules are pleasant tasting and happily sugar, salt and starch free. For breakfast I sometimes take two tablespoons of these granules along with raw wheat germ and brewers yeast and raw sunflower and pumpkin seeds on my sugarfree granola or oats with low fat yogurt and berries. These healthful granules can also be used in soups, salads and juices. (Approximately $13 per 16 oz. can.)

Shiitake

These mushrooms from Japan (now starting to be culti-vated here) are a delicacy, but can also produce interferon and have been reported in Japan as being effective in treat-ing cancer. In China they have been rated number one for giving one eternal youth and longevity.

Along with being delicious, they prevent high blood pres-sure and heart disease, tend to lower cholesterol, build resis-tance against viruses and disease, and help overcome fatigue and re-vitalize the organism.

Wheatgrass

Dr. Ann Wigmore of the Hippocrates Institute in Boston, Mass., has popularized wheatgrass and claims it is the richest of all foods and contains the largest amounts of enzymes (it is raw, remember), vitamins, minerals, and trace elements. Dr. Wigmore reports that wheatgrass therapy, along with raw living food, has helped her patients eliminate cancer, heart problems and many other disorders including mental health problems. You can sprout your own organic wheatgrass in trays along with other sprouts, and put them in a salad with raw carrots, onions, apple, shiitake, lecithin and raw seeds and nuts with a dressing of low fat yogurt or just flax oil and cider vinegar. My mouth is watering already!

The raw living food diet (see appendix on enzymes) should be included as much as possible in a healthy way of eating. In New York City Dr. Dian Griesel is an exponent of this Natural Hygiene philosophy. She asserts that vegetarianism is the correct diet for humans since we are constitutionally adapted to a diet of fruits, vegetables, nuts and seeds eaten in compatible combinations in their raw natural state. Mankind's similarity physiologically to the vegetarian primates and stark contrast to the meat eating carnivores is made clear.

Her Health and Nutrition Report is informative and a breath of fresh air. If you get confused about meat or no meat, dairy or no dairy, raw or cooked foods and various supplements, ask a friend to help you find *your* answer through kinesiology (muscle testing as described earlier) and by observing your own reactions to different foods. You may also wish to have a nutritional physician test you for food allergies.

Personally I feel great on the high enzyme, high fiber, high sprouted seeds and grains raw living food way, (no wonder I feel *high*). In the cold season I add soups, lightly steamed vegetables, sea foods, occasionally fertilized eggs, (roosters are part of the Great Design too) and since even the organic foods one buys may not be up to par, I also include many of these supplements along with the other "miracle foods." As long as my tennis and tango continue to improve I plan to stay with it!

Vitamin F — Essential Fatty Acids

Also known as polyunsaturates, these acids are not made by the body and must be supplied through diet. Along with flax oil which has already been eulogized, this important linoleic acid is also found in many vegetables and vegetable oils. But beware! If such oils are heated (that old nemisis again) or processed, linoleix acid is converted to undesirable trans fatty acids. If you eat fish, salmon and mackerel are the best sources of fatty acids, and black currant and primrose and borage oil are also excellent sources.

These goodies aid in preventing as well as alleviating arthritis, lowering blood pressure, lowering cholesterol levels, reducing the rate of breast cancer, candidiasis, (yeast overgrowth), coronary heart disease, and blood clot formation. Research in Oregon University and in Japan concur that a deficiency of these essential fatty acids leads to impaired recall. If this is a problem with you, might you be ready for an oil change?

Ginseng

This remarkable herb has long been used in the Orient as the king of all tonics. The Native Americans also used it for general healing purposes, and Russian scientists claim that it improves glandular function, has a positive effect on the sex glands, improves physical and mental activity and helps overcome fatigue by increasing the use of fatty acids as an energy source. If you buy this supplement, make sure there is no sugar or added coloring.

According to James Balch, M.D., ginseng can be used for impotence, stress, energy, cocaine withdrawal, diabetes, radiation protection, colds and chest problems. It enhances immune function, stimulates the appetite and normalizes blood pressure.

Coenzyme Q10

Twelve million people in Japan alone take this nutrient daily. It is found in every cell and is necessary for the cell to do its work. Due to bad diet, stress, and lack of exercise, deficiences occur. Research studies show that it strengthens the cardiovascular system, re-vitalizes the body's natural defense system, energizes cells and increases endurance and normalizes blood pressure.

Along with the amino acid L-taurine, it is of great value in preventing and curing congestive heart failure. In a study reported in the *Japanese Circulation Journal,* 3 grams of taurine daily were found to be more effective than 30 mg. of CoQ10.

The combination of 30 mg. of CoQ10 four times a day and one gram of taurine three times a day yields significant improvement in cardiac output, shortness of breath, palpitation and edema.

Anti-Oxidants

This popular word describes a group of vitamins, minerals and enzymes that help protect our body from the formation of free radicals. Now free radicals, another word you will be hearing more and more, are atoms with unpaired electrons seeking to grab on to other molecules, and in so doing cause damage to cells, impair our immune system, and lead to infections and various degenerative diseases.

Obviously such friends we are better off without. They have always been a part of the life process, and result for example from the natural process of food digestion. But here's the rub. We are being overwhelmed by them because in our unhealthy world and life styles, they are created by cigarette smoke, radiation, the plethora of toxic chemicals that are in our food, air and water, and the effects of over-exposure to the sun's rays.

Cholesterol has been getting bad press these days, even though it is a necessary and important substance that is a major constituent of our bodies and forms 50% of our cell membranes. Here again balance—the Greeks called it the golden mean—is the key. A normal cholesterol level is between 180 and 220. Above or below is not desirable. The "good" HDL cholesterol is protective of the heart, but the "bad" LDL when affected by free radicals, forms part of the plaque that can lodge in the vascular walls (remember the article by Rath and Pauling referred to earlier, "Solution to the Puzzle of Human Cardiovascular Disease").

The answer, then, to keeping a healthy heart and avoid-ing the number one killer of our era, is to keep one's choles-terol down within normal limits, avoid tobacco and other toxins in food (get organic food or raise it and sprout it yourself, procure pure water, and move to places that have air fit to breathe if possible.

You can also bolster your inner troops against the swarm-ing free radical enemies by sending in daily reenforcements of—you guessed it—anti-oxidants. Avant-garde nutrition-ally oriented physicians in New York City like Dr. Azim Etemade, Dr. Robert C. Atkins and Dr. Robert Wallis all recommend such supplementation.

A sensible basic program would include four or five grams of vitamin C per day. Note that C, which we have stated is not produced by humans, both protects the vascular walls as well as destroys free radicals. If this is not a good buy, I do not know what is. I also recommend vitamin E—eight to

1200 units a day. Many studies have shown its heart benefits, in particular the Harvard Nurses study which came out
in November of 1992. Of 87,000 female nurses in this part of
the study, 17% took vitamin E supplements. After eight
years of follow up, it was found that women who had taken
vitamin E for more than two years had a 46% lower risk of
suffering a heart attack! As an added bonus, there are no
noxious side effects (iatrogenic) with E.

Beta carotene is also recommended; 25,000 units per day
for vitamin A activity. Dr. Robert Atkins mentions a study
in the mid-eighties which showed a 50% drop in heart
attacks among men who used this supplement. Selenium,
also recommended, is a powerful anti-oxidant that works
with vitamin E and protects the immune system from free
radicals. It also has been linked to being protective against
both cancer and heart disease. On hundred mg a day are
recommended. These big four, along with our prudent diet,
exercise and meditation techniques should let you sleep easier, and even celebrate your hundredth birthday.

One added note regarding heart disease. Before you opt
for surgery investigate *chelation,* which has worked wonders
with hundreds of thousands of people. Your wholistic
physician (see the list in the back of this book if necessary)
will inform you further.

Believe it or not, the leopard has changed its spots! At
long last, the orthodox medical community is finally recom-
mending antioxidant supplements as a means of preventing
as well as treating disease!

The ultra-conservative *Journal of the American Medical
Association* recommended "vitamin supplements" as a way of
preventing heart disease. (JAMA August 19, 1992, pp. 871-
877.) Another study reported in the May 1992 issue of the
journal *Epidemiology* showed that vitamin C could increase

the average lifespan of men by six years! So now not only will your prudence and self management be rewarded, but you may also enjoy the blessings of orthodoxy as well!

You will enjoy the following results of my miracle food regimen:

- You will lose excess weight and fat.
- You will feel lighter and brighter.
- You will have more sustained energy.
- You will feel better about life, yourself, and others.
- Your blood pressure should reach a healthier level.
- Your HDL (good cholesterol) will increase.
- Your low-density lipoprotein (LDL, the bad cholesterol) should decrease.
- Your self-esteem will grow as you take charge of your life.
- You will be ready and able to improve the rest of your life.
- You will be a kinder person to yourself and others.
- Your thoughts will be more positive as you feel more alive.
- Feeling happier, you will be more grateful to the Higher Power and grow spiritually.
- You will have preventive insurance against free radical damage to DNA and cancer.
- You will have preventive insurance against diabetes, stroke, and cardiovascular disease.
- Foods as medicine will help you avoid iatrogenic disease.

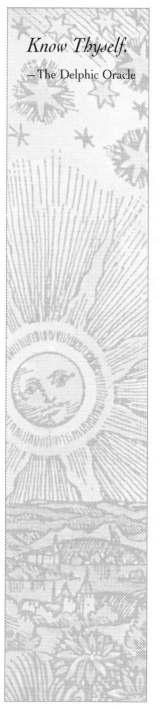

APPENDIX IV

Syntonic Education — Developing the Whole Person

As important as it is to help alleviate the suffering of human beings, and as gratifying as this can be (for myself as a wholistic psychotherapist and for other practitioners), it is far more important to use our knowledge to *prevent* emotional illness. While we are helping one person regain wholesomeness and self-respect, hundreds and thousands of others are being damaged in an emotional plague of such proportions that no person is untouched by it. The majority of people in our society

331

are severely crippled in their ability to be physically relaxed, emotionally positive and assertive, mentally clear and constructive, and spiritually in tune with the Life Force. In vital and free people, the stream of life flows easily and pleasurably; they are therefore life positive: *for* themselves, *for* others, and for life itself. Such people discover the meaning of life in fully living it, enthusiastically and creatively. As Helen Keller said, "Life is an adventure or it is nothing."

For most people in our society, the life stream becomes dammed up in infancy and early childhood. The work of Spitz with infants has shown how severely the natural functions of trust and love can be damaged when the infant is deprived of sufficient warmth, love, and bodily contact. Harlow's research with young primates has also demonstrated the need of bodily closeness with the mother and the emotional, sexual, and behavioral disturbances that occur in later life when this need is not satisfied. The natural law that developed over millions of years of evolutionary process clearly indicates that mother and infant should be together from birth until weaning, which in natural circumstances—primarily, as we have seen, in happy "primitive" societies—occurs when the infant is between one and two years of age. Although the science of psychology has made clear the crucial importance of the earliest years on the personality, custom and technology in so-called civilized societies begin to disrupt the natural order of things literally at birth; (See Dr. LeBoyer's great book *Birth without Violence.*)[1] and even before![2]

Consequently, modern humans are suffering from a basic

---

[1] F. LeBoyer, *Birth Without Violence,* Alfred Knopf, N.Y., 1980.

[2] T. Verny, *The Secret Life of the Unborn Child,* Dell Pub., N.Y., 1981.

anxiety, an underlying and constant state of fear that distorts their well-being and natural capacity for rationality. When the root is damaged, the tree is maimed and never grows to its full potential. When this crippling occurs in the foundation stage of the personality, the person becomes more vulnerable to other stresses at all the later stages of development. For this reason, it is often necessary to go back and resolve experiences that remain to disturb the well-being and damage the wholeness of the person. Such early violations of the natural order create disturbed and negative emotions, which are further aggravated by destructive experiences in families and schools.

Even well-meaning parents and educators rarely know how to protect and nourish the child's health and happiness, and they tend to repeat the mistakes of the past. Faulty nutrition; lack of communication, empathy, and respect; negative instead of positive discipline; and the suppression of feelings prevail. Toxicity, glandular disturbances, and physical illness aggravate emotional instability, tension, and disease—and vice versa—with the result that a vicious circle of disturbance is set in motion. This, in turn, is accompanied by irrational thinking and mental illness, in another vicious circle. An inefficient social system that does not offer employment for everyone who wants to work and be self-supporting compounds the problem, and universal physical, emotional, mental, and spiritual illness is the outcome. Like past civilizations, we shall have to adapt or perish.

The symptoms of this mass illness are appearing earlier due to the permissive attitudes of society. Crime, drug addiction, violence, venereal disease, and unwanted pregnancy are increasing among adolescents. The need is not for repression, even if that were possible. The dam is broken. Our challenge now is to rechannel the flood waters in constructive directions, through the kind of authentic education and group reeducation that can foster self-respect, personality integration, emotional security, constructive self-discipline, rational thinking, and positive assertiveness for oneself and for needed changes in society.

We have enough knowledge of the nutritional, physical, emotional, and mental requirements for health, as well as educational methods and group dynamic procedures to implement this knowledge. Perhaps the disturbed inner state and open violence so common among our youth will force us to overcome our inertia and fear of change. In view of the problems to be dealt with, it seems to me that a program such as the one I outline in this appendix is a bare minimum. If we were to follow it, society could save untold wealth—in precious lives and in resources that are now squandered in prisons and hospitals. Healthy and happy people enjoy doing good things for themselves and others and are spontaneously just and kind. On the other hand, the disturbed mind—twisted and driven by a toxic, tense body and negative emotions—becomes a diabolical force in society. Is not prevention wiser than cure, and education more desirable than punishment?

A prophetic voice has spoken out on this crucial issue of the behavior of our youth, the role of education and the fate of our great country and its democratic institutions. I refer to Walter H. Annenberg, who recently made a $500 million gift to public education to help support academic innovations in schools.[3]

This noble citizen, of great heart and mind, made the following statement: "I am deeply troubled by the violence in

---

[3] *The New York Times,* Dec. 18, 1993.

some grade schools and high schools, and if this continues, it will not only erode the educational system but will destroy our way of life in the United States." I am totally in accord with the import and wisdom of this statement.

To prevent this destructive behavior we must start at the beginning; birthing without violence and universal guidance for mothers with infants encouraging nursing which would give a secure foundation to each person. Guidance toward proper nutrition would strengthen the physical and mental health of the infant-child to avoid the sugar and junk foods that are undermining health. Then schools in which the hearts and feelings and the self-esteem of students are as important as knowledge would fulfill the true meaning of education. The Delphic Oracle has spoken!

When every school and college has a Department of Personal Growth and each student an opportunity to develop self-understanding, understanding of others, inner peace (by learning about proper nutrition and relaxation), and reverence of life, throughout their schooling, Mr. Annenberg's vision will be fulfilled.

The goal is to combat the emotional plague of tension, anxiety, and hostility that manifests itself in the vast misery of alcoholism, drug addiction, accidents, degenerative diseases, psychosomatic illness, crime, corruption, mental illness, prejudice, childhood neurosis, and the breakdown of the family.

The means to this goal are as follows:

1. Establish a Department of Personal Growth in every school and college. We have the skills to educate one-fourth of the teachers in grade school and high school as specialists in group discussion and group dynamics, so that students can learn to focus

on *themselves* as the subject matter. Such groups could help release negative emotions, use anger as a positive force for change, minimize negative attitudes toward the self and others, and help develop the self-knowledge, self-respect, and self-discipline that would lead to richer lives and healthier communities.

Students would learn the value of honest and constructive sharing of thoughts and feelings in an atmosphere of mutual respect and understanding, and the role of creative leadership. With these groups as a model, as future parents, students would develop the ability to communicate constructively and establish healthier and more democratic families, when they become parents, avoiding the destructive extremes of license and dictatorship that generally prevail.

Personal growth workshops with fifteen students and a group facilitator would meet twice per week for one hour per meeting. The effect of five or ten such pilot programs on the social, personal, and academic functioning of the students participating would be evaluated after one year.

2. Require, on the college level, workshops in personal growth and understanding so that a college degree would indicate a significant measure of self-awareness and growth in personal values and maturity, *as well as* academic knowledge. Knowledge is power, but driven by fear and hostility, it is a loose cannon on the deck.

   With trained group leaders in an atmosphere of openness and understanding, students would have the opportunity to discover and understand their feelings, change undesirable attitudes and behavior, clarify their values and goals, and free their energies for more productive and happier living. They would increase their skill and competence to be happier persons and future parents—the two most important human responsibilities that have been neglected by education!

3. Graduate schools in education and religion must educate students to become specialists in counseling and in personality growth, so that all classrooms, community centers, and religious institutions would offer competent guidance to persons who need help to cope with the emotional stresses of living. Such trained leaders could also help children and adults find more intensive care from other specialists when necessary. When a colleague and I started such groups at New York University for graduate students in education and human relations, students judged this to be *the most important and valuable experience in their whole education.*[4] They became aware that the values of quality living and growth, self-understanding, self-expression, self-respect, and understanding other persons were more important than all the academic information they had acquired. We forget that a large portion of academic knowledge is forgotten and never used.

---

[4] H. Giles and R. Kronemeyer, "Self-evaluation of a Group Therapy Experience by Graduate Students and Its Implications," *The International Journal of Social Psychiatry,* Vol. XI, No. 3, 1965.

Eleven Ways to Strengthen the Goodness in Human Nature

Every person has emotional problems to a lesser or greater extent. Without help, such difficulties usually worsen rather than disappear. Inner tension and confusion create problems in relations with other people which often generate frustration, resentment, and—eventually—hopelessness and despair. Too often secrecy and shame are connected with anxiety, guilt, hostility, and sexuality—the raw materials of inner conflicts. With a trained leader-facilitator in required school and college personal growth groups, the following factors aid the process of personal growth in a group setting:

1. In a group, one is joined with others in the common goal of finding more satisfying ways of living. Whether child or adult, facing one's fears and problems in an atmosphere of mutual respect and shared honesty and encouragement can be crucial. Not only can alienation be overcome, but hope and strength can be liberated and directed toward healthy and productive goals. The periods of childhood and adolescence can be turning points toward negative or positive ways of being and *lifelong* behavior patterns.

2. In a group where honesty is valued, troublesome feelings that have been buried can be brought to awareness and dealt with. Anxieties and guilt feelings, stemming from irrational influences in childhood, cause us to hide emotions even from ourselves. Often we are only aware of the symptoms that arise from such tension and stress:

depressed feelings, panic states, vague anxiety, self-destructive or violent behavior, and a variety of psychosomatic ailments. I would estimate that such ailments comprise as much as 80 percent of all symptoms for which people seek help. The constructive rechanneling of such vast misdirected energies, against oneself and others, is surely a responsibility of genuine education. If the group process which encourages honest communication is "the greatest invention of the twentieth century" (Carl Rogers), the task is to make such growth experience available to all children and adults in our society!

3. The expression of one's true feelings is helped by interaction and communication with others, who also learn to risk honest self-expression. Freer members can blaze the trial for others who are more blocked in their ability to express themselves. The catharsis of negative feelings in an atmosphere of acceptance can liberate tensions that would otherwise be acted out in destructive and antisocial behavior. Such relief minimizes the anxiety, guilt, and hostility which plague individuals of all ages in our society.

4. The source of negative feelings and the irrational ideas that maintain them can be explored and challenged in group discussion. It is common experience that as negative feelings are released and understood and the unrealistic ideas that accompany them are examined, new ways of feeling, thinking, and positive emotions develop as mutual understanding, self-respect, and respect for others are encouraged.

5. Through creative group communication, members learn how to help themselves and how to understand and help others as well. Both children and adults develop keen awareness of negative lifestyles and characteristic behavior patterns in other group members (such as self-negation, belligerence, passivity, insincerity, withdrawal, excessive dependence, and lack of self-worth). Their honest reactions to such self-defeating ways of thinking and feeling often evoke emotional responses and gradual insight that are essential to inner and outer growth. As persons gradually change their self-defeating attitudes and help others do the same, they increase their understanding and respect for *themselves* as well as others.

6. In a group, with the support of other individuals, one tends to see the leader more realistically than in the greater dependency of the one-to-one relationship in individual therapy. In private counseling the individual is at the counselor's mercy. As a fallible human with his or her own neurotic tendencies, the counselor may tend to be passive, aloof, overconcerned, dictatorial, or unstable. Often people who have valid reactions to the counselor's difficulties are told that it is their distortion. This is less likely to happen when other individuals give their reactions to the group leader, which helps participating members strengthen their own judgment and mature to a sense of equal worth in relation to the leader.

7. Seeing others improve and change encourages group members to deal with their own remaining problems. The struggle to change deeply set pat-

terns can be a long, lonely, and discouraging road. The obstacles to getting free from inner fears, guilts, and irrational thoughts must be faced and not avoided. And since we imperfect humans tend toward avoidance because it is easier at the moment (though it leads to long-range extended suffering), the prodding and encouragement from others can be invaluable.

8. Emotional difficulties always manifest themselves in relation to others, as well as to oneself. In the original group, the family, some or all of the conditions for healthy personality growth are usually lacking. How could this be otherwise, since education for parenthood is practically nonexistent? In an atmosphere created by a warm, understanding leader (a substitute parent figure), the new "group family" is usually tender on real feelings and a genuine need for help, and tough on rigidity, artificiality, and negativity. These patterns are not merely discussed and analyzed; they are experienced and brought into sharp focus as they occur. Thus childish and destructive conditioning can be challenged, understood, and changed in actual relationships.

9. Contrary to popular opinion, specific areas of emotional problems can be reached and helped in reeducational groups. Individuals vary in their ability to face and explore different problem areas: hostility, dependence, guilt, sexuality, grandiosity, prejudice, self-negation, perfectionism, and fear of risking, growing, and loving. Seeing others feel and gradually overcome their anxiety, sadness, hopelessness, and suppressed

aggression helps other group members deal with
their particular problem areas that thwart productivity and happiness.

10. The group process of honest communication
encourages the growth of healthy independence
and positive self-assertion. In the group, as a second "family," the damaging influences of the original family (real, imaginary, or exaggerated) can be
uncovered and resolved. Since the individual
develops strength and assertiveness in relation to
many other persons, there is less dependency on
one person and growing confidence in one's own
resources. The experience of being accepted in
honest relationships carries over into other relationships after the group experience, and the freedom and dignity that go with being an authentic
person are strengthened.

11. The group whose purpose is personal growth fur-
thers healthy ways of feeling, thinking, and relating. Becoming freer and more alive involves not
only the release and resolution of past and present
negative emotional patterns that are isolating and
destructive. It also involves learning pleasurable
and creative ways of feeling, thinking, behaving,
and relaxing. As fear and tension lessen, pleasure
and affection increase: Members gradually change
from feeling artificial to feeling real; from a feeling
of isolation to a feeling of belonging; from feeling
guilty to feeling self-respect; from feeling dependent to feeling self-confident; from hostility to positive self-assertion; from false pride to self-esteem;
from dis-ease toward ease and well-being. Pent-up
emotions that have either simmered inwardly or

exploded outwardly gradually change to a more balanced flow of feelings. The group is ideal soil for tender shoots of emotions and behavior before they are transplanted into the more difficult outside world. However, those who are too disturbed to grow in a group setting can be referred for help before they act out their problems on society.

The basic emotional education of the person occurs in families and schools. Rarely are the conditions met which safeguard and nourish the healthy growth of the person toward emotional and social maturity: honest communication, warmth, dependability, tenderness, and respectful caring for oneself and others (known as love). What is usually called love so often lacks the essential ingredient, respect. Only in those rare human families in which reason is combined with positive emotions can one see the real human potential for mental and emotional health. Such a state is not merely an absence of symptoms; it is a quality of aliveness that enables one to function in work and love as a whole person, to face the problems of living with reasonableness and courage, and to respect one's own life, the lives of others, and life itself. Such families will continue to be the exception as long as there is a paucity of education for emotional growth in our schools and colleges. Actually experiencing emotional growth and democratic leadership in personal growth workshops will give students a healthy model that they can use as they become parents to create a more wholesome life for their children.

Many centuries before the West emerged from the Dark Ages and undertook the Promethean task of conquering nature, the East was launching its astronauts in the inner universe to explore humankind's psyche and spirit. In India, yoga (union) developed a wholistic view of mankind, the "featherless biped." In China, Taoism (The Way) explored the energy pathways of the *chi* (the Life Force); and in Japan the flowering was manifested in aikido (the way of harmony with the Life Force or Ki).

The techniques of these great disciplines can be taught in schools at the end of each Personal Growth Group to teach deep and serene respiration, physical relaxation, body-mind unity, quieting the mind at will (to discover the ability to think or not think is Enlightenment), experiencing Oneness with the Life Force as the ultimate source of authentic self-esteem, and using affirmations and visualizations to fortify the Self.

Knowledge of healthy nutrition is also essential for physical, emotional, mental, and spiritual health—and the prevention of cancer and heart disease. Ironically, "modern" medicine has yet to understand the teaching of Hippocrates: "Let your food be your medicine."

Pulling the weeds and cultivating the flowers are both essential for effective personality change and growth. Only the best of the East and West is worthy of our youth and of our country. For the first time in the history of the human race, we can break the chain of generations of victims. Then we shall make a giant step for mankind, of greater significance than the vaunted first step on the moon. Only those with self-knowledge, self-respect, and self-control can enjoy freedom. And "justice for all," if it be more than a lofty phrase, can only be built on the bedrock of self-respect and reverence for life. Without these attitudes that stem from a unity of heart and mind, life is "solitary, poor, nasty, brutish and short" as Thomas Hobbes opined in *The Leviathan*. Now is the time to focus on creating not merely knowledgeable but also "good" people. Marcus Aurelius put it best: "The good man acts the same, whether there are laws or not."

Let us put ancient wisdom into action. The wisest words ever spoken would support the crucial and central importance of personal growth groups: the Delphic Oracle counseled, "Know Thyself." And with a similar depth of insight, Socrates said, "The unexamined life is not worth living."

The alternative is stark: for either way we go we shall reap what we have sown. Our contemporary prophets, the seers and poets of our time, penetrate to the marrow of the problem: the choice between true education and catastrophe. My friend Karen Singh, the contemporary Indian mystic and philosopher, thunders "We have to transit to complementarity in place of competition, convergence in place of conflict, wholism in place of hedonism . . . we must heal the split within the human psyche."

W. H. Auden warns in no uncertain terms, "We are lecturing on navigation while the ship is going down." This is a penetrating description of our head-centered education, which has forgotten the whole Self (see the Personality Chart), failed to remember that "out of the heart are the issues of life," neglected the spirit that alone gives nobility to mankind, and sends endless droves of compassionless moral pygmies into the world to participate in the rat race of acquisitiveness.

Untold millions of our youth are conditioned to be chronically trapped in the fight-or-flight mode, which creates unending anxiety and conflicting impulses to run, to attack, and/or to submit. The purpose of all therapies and religions is to help humans attain the parasympathetic state of serenity and syntony in which alone there is "the peace that passeth understanding."

Pascal knew this when he wrote, "the trouble with Western man is that he cannot spend five minutes quietly in an empty room." This misguided emergency system, nature's gift for survival in the face of genuine threats to one's life, triggers the plethora of addictions that flesh is heir to in our Age of Anxiety. Seeking the "easy" way of immediate relief and gratification, and ignoring the rigorous truth that would "set one free," the hapless addict wastes his or her resources and compounds woe. In such a state, the lie takes ascendancy, honor is cast aside, self-respect is sold for a tuppence, decency is abrogated, compassion for self and others is nullified, the law of the jungle prevails, and the seven deadly sins have a field day.

The Genghis Khans of our century, Adolph Hitler and Josef Stalin, were once schoolboys. Though they matriculated academically, their inner spiritual emptiness, hatred, and worthlessness mushroomed into a mammoth and insatiable addiction to power. Their successors are sitting in classrooms today. Hopefully there will be personal growth workshops in which they will be guided to regain the Self that was their birthright.

The three R's are important, but cultivating the fourth R—Respect for self, for others, and for life itself—is long overdue and imperative. Cultivating the healthy positive Self in each person would save and vitalize the American dream—the "land of the free and home of the brave."

> *Happiness is the norm. One can cure depression but not enthusiasm.*

Overcoming Depression Without Dangerous Drugs

Depression has many causes, and the Syntonic or total approach looks at all of them. Viral syndromes like Epstein Barr can undermine the energy of the body, as can an overgrowth of yeast (known as candidiasis) from past use of antibiotics. Environmental and food allergies can also wreak havoc on the system and create depression and irritability.

Another important area to examine is the food you eat. The neurotransmitters dopamine, seratonin, and

347

norephinephrine regulate behavior and the way you feel. A meal high in saturated fat will depress the production of neurotransmitters, whereas a vegetarian meal, broiled salmon, or a large salad will have an uplifting effect. Here, too, remember the symptoms that go with eating refined sugar—"the sugar blues." Also remember that sugar depletes the vitamin B stores of the body, which are crucial to the functioning of the nervous system. Take a tablespoon of brewer's yeast each day—the best source of vitamin B—with your cereal.

Thyroid malfunction can also cause lethargy, overweight, and depression. A nutritionally-oriented physician can test your thyroid, which regulates metabolism and hormone production.

The usual psychiatric approach to treating depression is with drugs; currently the favorite is Prozac. Psychiatrists may ignore or be unaware of the aforementioned culprits; patients will be given Prozac (which has been cited for 23,067 adverse drug reactions, including 1,436 suicide attempts and 1,313 deaths). Happily there are better, drugless ways.

Exercise is a safe and effective mood elevator. It stimulates endorphins in the brain, which create a sense of well-being without the agitation caused by Prozac. A study at the University of New Mexico revealed that sedentary middle-aged men were more depressed and had lower levels of endorphins than more active men.

A healthy low-fat and low-protein diet of fruit, whole grains, vegetables (raw or steamed lightly), seafood, and raw nuts and seeds is essential for general well-being. A formerly depressed patient told me that since he was on this diet (along with psyllium powder every day to clean the colon), and exercising, his mood was always bright and alive. As we have seen, supplements of vitamins C, E A, B complex (plus brewer's yeast); the minerals magnesium, zinc, and selenium; and fish oil capsules are also important. Herbs can also help elevate energy, mood, and well-being. One herb commonly used in Europe as an anti-depressant is Saint-John's-wort, which has been shown to increase dopamine production in the brain. Ginkgo biloba has also been effective in improving mood, sociability, reaction time, and circulation.

Psychogenic depression can be caused by negative relationships and repressed anger. Often hapless couples either do not talk, or fight when they do. I have seen the empathy exercise (see Appendix II) enable couples to heal their shared depression, increase their self-respect and respect for each other, and enjoy much greater well-being.

Overreacting to life's disappointments can throw one into depression and negativity in thought, feeling, and behavior. Using Syntonic techniques such as challenging such thoughts and mobilizing the power of positive anger (pounding, stamping, yelling) and integrating thought, feeling, and movement through centering and visualization can also get the stream of life flowing positively again.

Spiritual resources are also available to overcome negativity and depression. "The Lord is the Spirit, and where the Spirit of the Lord is, there is freedom." (II Corinthians 3:17) Prayer and meditation can lift our spirits, help us contact the Higher Power, free us from egocentricity, encourage us to give to others, and liberate the love in our hearts that can cast our fear and depression.

The Syntonic Way to Kick the Blues

Before you see a doctor, do the following things for yourself:

1. Make sure your diet is healthy and free of saturated fat, refined sugar, bleached flour, sodas, etc., and take supplements as recommended.
2. If you suspect environmental or food allergies, use kinesiology or the elimination diet to check out these items.
3. Make sure you exercise every day, even if you would rather be a couch potato.
4. Try the herbs mentioned on page 349. Take one or two droppers of Saint-John's-wort extract three times daily in water on an empty stomach. Also try three capsules of ginkgo three times a day, and Ginseng as well. To help sleep take valerian and also chamomile tea.
5. Use the empathy exercise on page 305 if you are in a negative relationship. If your partner is unwilling, decide whether you want to remain with such a negative person.
6. Use the self-help techniques described in chapters 7 and 8 to break out of negative thoughts, feelings, and behavior, and strengthen the healthy (parasympathetic) state as described in the Personality Chart as the healthy Self.
7. Call on the Life Force that created you with the prayer of Saint Augustine: "Lord give me the strength to change what I cannot accept, accept what I cannot change, and the wisdom to distinguish between the two." Use the aikido method to relax your body and send your energy out toward the world in positive ways, so you regain harmony with the universe.
8. If you still are not positive and in tune with life, find a nutritionally-oriented physician to determine if

there are viral problems, allergies, or thyroid malfunction that need further help.

Enzymes: The Missing Link?

It is possible to do everything right such as eating natural
whole organic foods, taking supplements (vitamins, herbs
and minerals) along with a healthy lifestyle, and still not
achieve the vitality that accompanies true health! The
answer lies in the fact that it is not only what you eat but
what you assimilate that counts!

The work of Dr. Edward Howell is fascinating in this
regard.[1] Enzymes are substances that make life possible,
and are involved in every chemical reaction that takes place
in the body. There are three different classes of enzymes;
metabolic enzymes that run our bodies, digestive enzymes
that digest our food, and food enzymes from raw food,
which start food digestion. Dr. Howell states that "our bodies—all our organs and tissues—are run by metabolic
enzymes. These enzyme workers take proteins, fats and carbohydrates (starches, sugars, etc.) and structure them into
healthy bodies, keeping everything working properly.
Every organ and tissue has its own particular metabolic
enzymes to do specialized work. No one has ever investi-
gated how many specific enzymes are needed to run the
heart, brain, lungs, kidneys, etc."

We are confronted here with an awesome facet of creation when you consider the trillions of cells which compose
the temple of the Spirit, the human body. If proper food is

---

[1] Dr. Edward Howell, *Enzyme Nutrition — The Food Enzyme Concept.* Avery
Publishing Group Inc. Wayne, N.J., 1985.

utilized by the uncanny intelligence of these enzymes, "keeping everything working properly," not only an absence of illness but radiant health ensues. But this is not the case! Instead of living vitally to a hundred years or more, and passing on when one's genetic clock runs out, most people are taken by the scourge of degenerative diseases long before their time.

There are two worms in the apple, friends. One of course is that our food is not raised organically in enzyme-rich and manure fertilized soil. Secondly, enzymes are destroyed by heat and cooking, as well as by canning! Originally mankind as a food gatherer ate raw fruits and vegetation. Today many of our fruits and vegetables look good but have been "fertilized" by synthetic fertilizers that were developed about fifty years ago. We are concerned with preserving the wolf and the eagle, but are still unaware of the enzyme, that microscopic life form upon which our existence and our health and longevity depend!

Eating cooked food primarily means that our bodies have to overwork to produce digestive enzymes. This diminishes the production of metabolic enzymes which are essential in the functioning of the blood, tissues and all the organs of the body. Raw foods contain their naturally occurring enzymes and therefore do not tax and deplete the body of its enzyme stores. For example, the Eskimo people on their raw food diet ate large amounts of fat that also was rich in lipase—the fat digesting enzyme. When they changed their lifestyle to canned milk and cooked food, white flour and sugar, they also fell into the torrent of degenerative diseases.

Dr. Howell also notes that before the age of pasteurized (heated) milk and its products, whole nations lived on raw milk, butter, cream and cheese which contained the enzyme lipase. Many of these people reached advanced age *without* developing cardiovascular disease. Could it be that raw milk contains something missing in the pasteurized product, which protects the body from the ravages of cholesterol, the same cholesterol that pasteurized milk and its products are reputed to inflict on its users?

I believe it is prudent, then, to eat as much of your food as possible organically grown, and raw. Also since you have been overdrawing your enzyme account for many years, start making deposits! (Remember the enzyme account can also be depleted by stress, injuries, negative thoughts, feelings and behavior (see the Personality Chart and the syntonic description of the healthy Self). As we lose our ability to assimilate our food, however healthy it may be, we can no longer repair and regenerate our cells. This leads to degenerative diseases, premature aging, and Adios.

To take prudent action in this important area of health, I suggest that you contact The Staff of Life; 1-800-743-7531 and ask them to send you their informative material. They have a basic enzyme formula that my patients and I have found valuable along with a variety of other formulas including vitamins and minerals.

P.S. I would be remiss if I failed to mention one of the most enjoyable and therapeutic experiences we are blessed with: laughter!

As you continue to clean out and re-vitalize your body, re-program your emotions toward the positive (parasympathetic) orientation, train your mind to think rationally or not think (as you choose) and constantly strengthen your connection with God, you will become the *good-natured person* you are meant to be in your natural healthy state.

I find, as I continue to work on myself and change and grow, that smiling energy and warm hearted laughter are more and more a part of my life and my fun in sharing humor with others. My friend Pila, a contemporary Hawaiian sage, says that in their tradition the wise men or Kahunas teach that we are all children, some wrinkled and some not, so playing is a must for everyone. We are all children playing on the sand, while before us lies the ocean of truth. So don't forget the elf in Self. Ecclesiastes reminds us that "there is a time for laughter" (3:4) and in Judges 19:6 it is written:

"Let thine heart be merry."

Godspeed

BIBLIOGRAPHY

Atkins, Robert C. *Dr. Atkins New Diet Revolution.* New York: M. Evans and Co., Inc. N.Y. 1992.

Anderson, Mary. *Colour Therapy: Healing with Color.* Calcutta, India: Firma LKM, Private Ltd., 1964.

Baba, Sai. *The Teachings of Sri Satya Sai Baba.* Tustin, CA: Pub. Book Center.

Bach, Edward. *Heal Thyself: An Explanation of the Real Cause and Cure of Disease.* London: The C. W. Daniel Co., Ltd., 1974.

Balch, James. *Prescription for Nutritional Healing.* New York: Avery Pub., 1990.

Beier, Ernst. *The Silent Language of Psychotherapy.* Chicago: Aldine, 1966.

Bible, King James version.

Bieler, Henry G. *Food Is Your Best Medicine.* Vintage Books, 1973.

Bricklin, Mark. *The Practical Encyclopedia of Natural Healing.* Rodale Press, 1976.

Burkitt, Denis, and Trowell, Hugh (Eds.). *Refined Carbohydrate Foods and Disease.* New York: Academic Press, 1975.

Capra, Fritjof. *The Tao of Physics.* Berkeley: Shambhala, 1975.

355

Cayce, Edgar. *On Diet and Health,* Hugh Lynn Cayce (Ed.). New York: Warner Books, 1969.

Chancellor, Philip. *Handbook of the Bach Flower Remedies.* London: C. W. Daniel Co., Ltd., 1971.

Chopra, Deepak. *Perfect Health.* New York: Harmony Books, 1991.

Cooper, Kenneth. *Aerobics.* New York: M. Evans and Co., Inc. 1968.

Davis, Adelle. *Let's Get Well.* New York: Harcourt Brace, 1965.

Epstein, Samuel. *The Politics of Cancer.* Sierra Book Club, 1978.

Feingold, Ben. *Why Your Child is Hyperactive.* New York: Random House, 1975.

Friedman, Meyer, and Rosenman, Ray. *Type A Behavior and Your Heart.* Fawcett, 1974.

Fromm, Erich. *The Art of Loving.* New York: Harper Colophon, 1956.

Gammon, Roland. *Nirvana Now.* New York: World Authors Ltd.

Gofman, John. *Poisoned Power.* Rodale Press, 1979.

Hoffman, Wendell. *Using Energy to Heal.* Ogden, UT: Private Pub.

Hrachovec, Josef. *Keeping Young and Living Longer.* Los Angeles: Sherbourne Press, 1972.

Johnson, Michael. *Eater's Digest: The Consumer's Factbook of Food Additives.* New York: Doubleday, 1972.

Kronemeyer, Robert. *Overcoming Homosexuality—Case Studies in Wholistic Therapy.* New York: Macmillan, 1979.

_____. "Syntonic Therapy: A Total Approach to the Treatment of Mental and Emotional Disturbances." *Psychotherapy: Theory, Research and Practice,* Fall 1977, Vol. 14, No. 3. pp. 249-262.

Kushi, Michio. *The Macrobiotic Way.* Avery Publishing Group, 1985.

Lappe, Frances Moore. *Diet for a Small Planet.* Ballantine Books, 1979.

LeBoyer, Frederick. *Birth without Violence.* New York: Knopf, 1978.

MacIvor, Virginia, and La Forest, Sandra. *Vibrations,* New York: S. Weiser, Inc.

May, Rollo, *Love and Will,* New York: W. W. Norton and Co., 1969.

Mead, Margaret. *Male and Female.* New York: William Morrow & Co., 1949.

Mendelsohn, Robert. *Confessions of a Medical Heretic.* Chicago: Contemporary Books, Inc., 1979.

Menninger, Karl. *Love Against Hate.* New York: Harcourt Brace, 1942.

Pauling, Linus. *Vitamin C and the Common Cold.* W. H. Freeman and Co., 1970.

Pelletier, Kenneth. *Mind as Healer, Mind as Slayer.* Dell, 1977.

Report on Organic Farming. Washington, DC: Office of Governmental and Public Affairs, U.S. Dept. of Agriculture.

Reuben, David. *The Save Your Life Diet.* New York: Ballantine Books, 1975.

Rowe, Albert. *Elimination Diets and the Patient's Allergies.* Philadelphia: Lea and Febiger, 1941.

Schroeder, Henry. *The Trade Elements and Man.* Devin-Adair Co., 1973.

Selye, Hans. *The Stress of Life.* New York: McGraw-Hill, 1976.

Shute, Wilfred. Complete, Updated Vitamin E Book. Keats, 1975.

Simonton, Carl. *Getting Well Again.* J. P. Tarcher, Inc., 1978.

Spino, Dyveke. *New Age Training for Fitness and Health.* New York: Grove Press, 1979.

Spitz, Rene. *The First Year of Life.* New York: International Universities Press, Inc., 1965.

Tagore, Rabindranath. *Gitanjali (Song Offerings)*. Boston: International Pocket Library, 1912.

Tansley, David. *Radionics and the Subtle Anatomy of Man*. England: Health Science Press, 1972.

Tompkins, Peter, and Bird, Christopher. *The Secret Life of Plants*. New York: Harper & Row, 1972; reprint, Avon Books, 1973.

Verney, Thomas. *The Secret Life of the Unborn Child*. New York: Dell Pub. Co., 1981.

Verrett, Jacqueline, and Carper, Jean. *Eating May Be Hazardous to Your Health*. New York: Simon & Schuster, 1974.

Williams, Roger. *The Wonderful World Within You*. New York: Bantam Books, 1977.

Yudkin, John. *Sweet and Dangerous*. Peter H. Wyden, Inc., 1972.

ABOUT THE AUTHOR

Dr. Robert Kronemeyer has gathered years of research, study, private practice and personal experience into one of the most thoroughly written books in the field of wholistic health practice. His wide range of educational studies and years of hands-on practical experience have resulted in a wholistic guidebook for well-being.

Dr. Kronemeyer studied philosophy at Amherst College, comparative religion at Union Seminary, and pre-medicine and clinical and social psychology at Columbia University. Other credits include post-doctoral work at the Psychiatric Institute, Bellevue Hospital, the Postgraduate Center for Psychotherapy, and the National Psychological Association for Psychoanalysis, where he became a senior analyst.

Always seeking a higher path to spiritual awareness himself, Kronemeyer has studied many disciplines and therapy techniques with world-renowned gurus and therapists. Gradually, he came to develop his own unique therapy, the integration of body, mind, emotions, and spirit that evolved into Syntonic Therapy, which he defines as integrating (syn) the energy vibrations (tonic) of the organism.

Individuals, as well as family groups can learn to communicate with themselves and others after utilizing Dr. Kronemeyer's simple techniques for self-renewal and self-healing.

Dr. Kronemeyer has presented lectures and workshops in universities in America as well as in India, Turkey, and Australia.

INDEX

A

Abkhasians, health status of, 21
addictive personality, 97-98
    and anxiety, 120-121
adversity, positive handling of,
    123, 203-5
affirmations
    for emotional health, 287-88
    lifetime affirmation, 290-91
    for personal growth, 287-88
agape, 150
aggressive types
    neurotic aggression, 227
    thought processes of, 167
    type A personality, 227-28
agnostics, 216, 262
aikido
    motto of, 243
    rules of, 244-46
    and transformation, 246
alcoholism, 56
alimentary massage, 74
allergies. *See* food allergies
Anderson, James, 41
anger, 125-26

and guilt, 125-26
as killer of love, 262
negative anger, effects of, 262
productive use of, 127, 134-35,
    141, 142-43, 262-63
animal products. *See* dairy
    products; meat
animals
    choice of foods by, 17
    fasting of, 16
Anaximander, 270
anti-oxidants
    benefits of, 327-29
    green tea as, 322
    recommended dosages,
        328-29
anxiety
    and addiction, 120-121
    as energy blockage, 122-23
anxious mind, 162
    characteristics of, 163-64
aphrodisiac herbs, 83, 87
appendicitis, 4, 27
Aristotle, 191
armoring, 164-65
arthritis, 4, 23-25

and psychological disturbance,
17-18, 37, 95-96
reflexology treatment of, 95-96
and sugar intake, 34-36

I

iatrogenic disease, 23, 78
Icarus, myth of, 247-48
imagery, use of positive imagery,
143-46
impotence, and diet, 82
indigestion, 27
indocin, 24
infertility, dietary
recommendations, 86
insomnia, solution to, 76-77
interferon, and shiitake
mushrooms, 324

J

James, William, 221
Jung, Carl, 238

K

karma, 76
kelp, 45
benefits of, 318-19
Kennel, John, 116
Ki, 74, 243-46, 271-72
kinesiology, 102-5
method in use of, 103
for music, 103
Klaus, Marshall, 116
kyolic, 316

L

lactic acid, negative effects of,
36-37

Leboyer, Frederick, 56, 200, 225
lecithin
benefits of, 323-24
in eggs, 43
legs, relaxation exercise for, 70, 72
Lewin, Kurt, 163, 295
Life Force, and breathing, 74
lifestyle, analysis of health
through, 11
lifetime affirmations, 290-91
Lippitt, Ronald, 295
loneliness, 121
and hostility, 226
love, 76, 147-51
agape, 150-51
and balance, 76
and body language, 149
capability to love, 225
and empathy, 259
eros, 149
false, motivations for, 148-49
fear of, 61, 234
feelings in, 61
genuine, characteristics of,
147-48
as opposite of fear, 280
philia, 150-51
and respect, 148-49, 222
spiritual aspects of, 256-58
low-density lipoproteins (LDL),
249, 323, 328
low-fat diet, percentage of fat in,
23
lunch, syntonic diet, 39
lung cancer, 97-98
lung disease, 4
lust, 222-26
case example, 223-26
and exploitation, 262
meaning of, 222, 261

Share the Magic of Chicken Soup

Chicken Soup for the Soul™
101 Stories to Open the Heart and Rekindle the Spirit

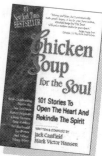

The #1 *New York Times* bestseller and ABBY award-winning inspirational book that has touched the lives of millions. Whether you buy it for yourself or as a gift to others, you're sure to enrich the lives of everyone around you with this affordable treasure.

Code 262X: Paperback $12.95
Code 2913: Hardcover $24.00
Code 3812: Large print $16.95

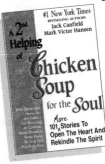

A 2nd Helping of Chicken Soup for the Soul™
101 More Stories to Open the Heart and Rekindle the Spirit

This rare sequel accomplishes the impossible—it is as tasty as the original, and still fat-free. If you enjoyed the first *Chicken Soup for the Soul,* be warned: it was merely the first course in an uplifting grand buffet. These stories will leave you satisfied and full of self-esteem, love and compassion.

Code 3316: Paperback $12.95
Code 3324: Hardcover $24.00
Code 3820: Large print $16.95

A 3rd Serving of Chicken Soup for the Soul™
101 More Stories to Open the Heart and Rekindle the Spirit

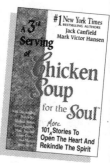

The latest addition to the *Chicken Soup for the Soul* series is guaranteed to put a smile in your heart. Learn through others the important lessons of love, parenting, forgiveness, hope and perseverance. This tasty literary stew will stay with you long after you've put the book down.

Code 3790: Paperback. $12.95
Code 3804: Hardcover. $24.00
Code 4002: Large print $16.95

Available at your favorite bookstore or call
1-800-441-5569 for Visa or MasterCard orders. Prices do not include shipping and handling. Your response code is BKS.